Cancer
in the Family

HELPING CHILDREN COPE WITH A PARENT'S ILLNESS

Sue P. Heiney, Ph.D., R.N.

Joan F. Hermann, M.S.W., L.S.W.

Katherine V. Bruss, Psy.D.

Joy L. Fincannon, R.N., M.S.

Published by
American Cancer Society
Health Content Products
1599 Clifton Road NE
Atlanta, Georgia 30329, USA
800-ACS-2345 (800-227-2345)
http://www.cancer.org

Printed in the United States of America

5 4 3 2 1   01 02 03 04 05

We gratefully acknowledge the use of some exercises adapted from *Kids Count, Too!* materials. Some of the original activities
were developed in 1996 by University of Minnesota Graduate, Michelle Ellefson, B.A., Patient Services Intern, Minnesota
Division, who created the workbook *Someone I Love Has Cancer.*

Library of Congress Cataloging-in-Publication Data

Cancer in the family: helping children cope with a parent's illness / Sue P. Heiney, ...[et al.].
     p. cm.
    Includes index.
     ISBN 0-944235-34-4
     1. Children of cancer patients. 2. Cancer--Patients--Family relationships. 3.
    Cancer--Psychological aspects. I. Heiney, Sue P. II. Title..

RC262.C29113 2001
362.1'96994--dc21

2001022090

Designed by
Shock Design, Inc., Atlanta, GA

Illustrations by
Chameleon Design, Atlanta, GA

Photography by
Billy Howard Photography, Atlanta, GA

A Note to the Reader
The information contained in this book is not intended as medical advice and should not be relied upon as a substitute
for consulting with your health care providers. All matters regarding your health require the supervision of professionals who are familiar with your physical and emotional needs. For more information contact your American Cancer
Society at 1-800-ACS-2345 (www.cancer.org).

Contributors

Lisa Jeannotte, M.A.
Writer/Editor
Health Communications Services
Atlanta, Georgia

Brenda Wagner, Ph.D.
Staff Psychologist
Children's Healthcare of Atlanta at
Scottish Rite
Atlanta, Georgia

Karen Dorshimer-Chaplin, M.Div.
Staff Chaplain
Spiritual Health Services
Fairview Southdale Hospital
Edina, Minnesota

Leslie Doehring, Psy.D.
Post–Doctoral Fellow
Children's Healthcare of Atlanta at
Scottish Rite
Atlanta, Georgia

MANAGING EDITOR
Katherine V. Bruss, Psy.D.

EDITORIAL REVIEW
Terri B. Ades, R.N., M.S., A.O.C.N.

PUBLISHING DIRECTOR
Emily Pualwan

PRODUCTION MANAGER
Candace Magee

Table of Contents

๛

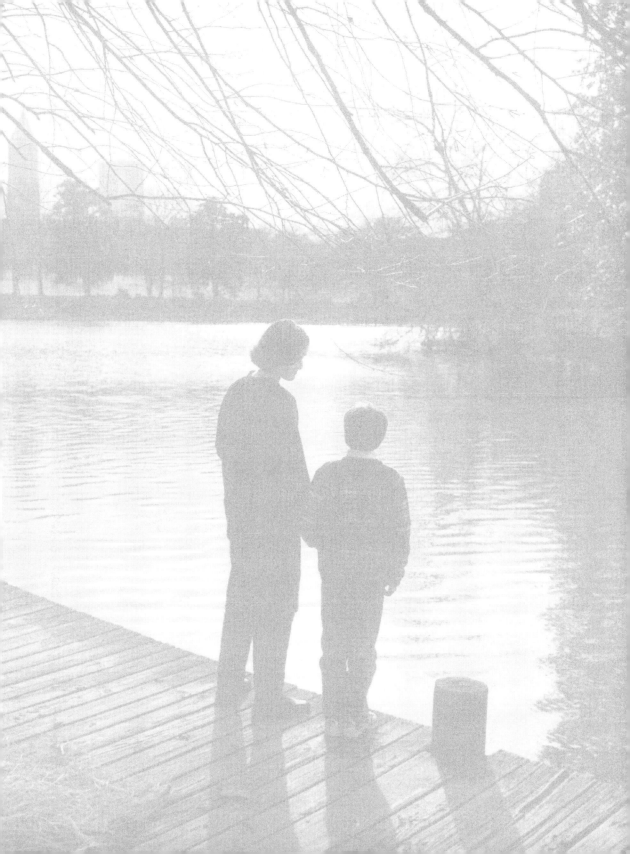

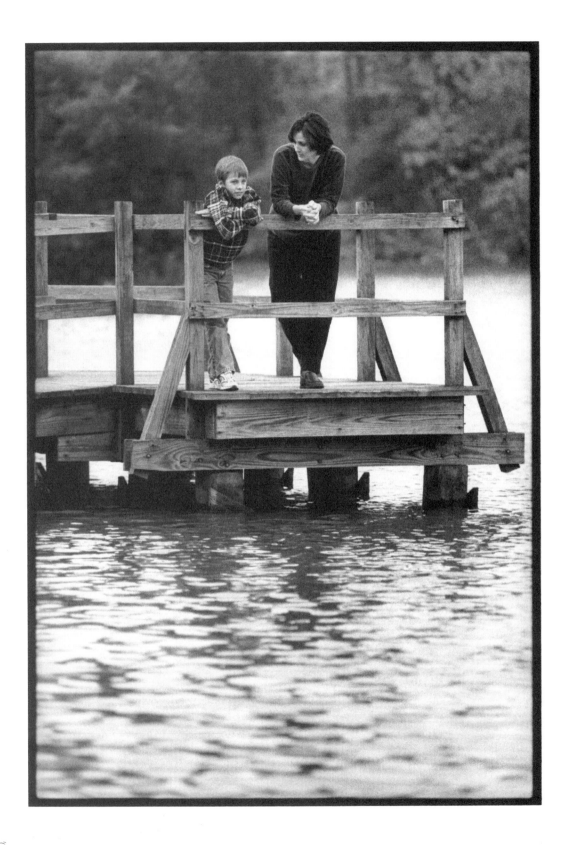

Introduction

৪৫

When you are a parent who has been diagnosed with cancer, your concerns are not only for yourself, but also for your children. Parents often ask themselves, "How will I be able to care for my children while I am going through all this?" There may be times when you have doubts about whether you can even take care of yourself. You may wonder how you are going to handle all of your parenting activities and responsibilities.

A diagnosis of cancer can be frightening not only to you, but also to your family. It is natural for families facing a new diagnosis of cancer to be upset and worried about how they will deal with this crisis in their lives. For families of young children or teens, these concerns may be greater as they wonder how their children will cope with the uncertainty a cancer diagnosis produces.

While there are many support groups for parents of children with cancer, resources are not as available for children whose parents have cancer. Medical teams are focused on treating the parents, so sometimes their children are left out of the picture. This book will help parents see through their children's eyes. Hands-on tools are included to guide parents through this difficult time. Concrete, practical suggestions highlight ways parents can help their children.

How Children Cope

It helps to understand how children react in many different circumstances so you'll know what to expect from your children. Of course each family has its own style of coping, but there are some basic principles that are universal.

Children Are Resilient

Parents know their children better than anyone else. They know what motivates them as well as what upsets them. They know how they usually react to bad news. Understanding children's reactions based on their ages and typical responses will help both parents and children through this difficult time. The best approach is to face things as they arise. If parents feel panicked or overwhelmed and ignore their children's behavior, the children may act out to get attention. So, it benefits everyone to deal with concerns up front.

Children respond well to simple words and honesty. Allowing them to express their feelings is also important. Getting them to do that can be somewhat difficult, especially when they are young. Just remember that they sometimes have more strength and insight than you ever imagined. As Erma Bombeck said about children and resiliency, "I have always believed that an army of fifteen two-year-olds could bring any enemy power to its knees in less than a day. But I never realized how resilient children are… Emotionally, they are like corks. Just when you think they are lost forever in the swirl of dark waters and rough seas, they surface to bob along awaiting the next storm."

One thing to be careful about is letting your own feelings be passed onto your children. It is better to find out what they are feeling. Then you can compare your feelings to theirs. Children need to know that many feelings are normal. They need help sorting out what they are feeling. Don't assume that your children feel exactly the same way you do.

Honesty Is the Best Policy

Children tend to accept what they are told at face value and they believe what you tell them. So, they need to be told the truth about what is happening in a straightforward manner (see Chapter 1). Protecting children from the truth can actually do more harm. If you try to keep big news a secret, children can sense something is happening anyway. They can pick up on unexpressed feelings or overhear others talking. For example, when a five-year-old daughter hears her mother on the telephone say, "Oh no," it is quite likely that she will be trying to figure out what is going on.

Children tend to imagine the worst, and they believe the world revolves around them. They think they have some kind of impact on all events in their lives, including a parent's cancer. The guilt that comes from this mistaken belief can be quite a burden. So, it is better to be honest about any situation that arises.

Children's Emotional Reactions to Crisis

There are several stages that children go through after hearing that their parent has been diagnosed with cancer. Not all children react the same way to distress, and each child adjusts on a different timetable. Common reactions are listed below. All of these can be normal responses to a crisis. If the reaction becomes prolonged or extreme, outside help will be needed (see Chapter 3).

Shock, Disbelief, and Denial

Although one would expect children to be shocked to hear news of their parent's illness, they often don't express shock in the same way as adults. Upon hearing bad news, young children typically do not gasp or make exclamations. Neither do teens, who pride themselves on keeping their cool. Instead, their first response may be to ask more questions. Or they may just be silent. The shock becomes real when a part of their lives must change; for example, when they don't get to play with a friend, or their dating schedules are curtailed for some reason.

Fear and Anxiety

When children's routines are disturbed and there is a general sense that "all is not well" within the home, they begin to have feelings of fear. Fear may be specific, such as fear of losing the parent. Anxiety is usually experienced as a more vague feeling of unrest and it is often not openly stated. Children may act differently or be more demanding when they are feeling anxious. Fears are often expressed in those quiet moments like just before bed. This is when children have the time and space to figure out how to express some of their feelings. Parents can help them recognize their feelings. Sometimes worries are expressed in play. Children may play pretend using stuffed animals or dolls. If parents listen and watch, they will see their children's inner world and learn much about their children's feelings.

Sadness

Feeling sad and down are normal feelings when facing changes related to a parent's illness. There are all kinds of sources for the sadness. For example, children may feel unhappy about the changes and losses the illness brings. Seeing their parents' sadness can also stir up feelings of sadness within them. But the most important things to do are to make sure the sadness is noted, expressed, and addressed. Depression will be explained in more depth when discussing potential warning signs and reasons for getting outside help or referrals (see Chapter 3).

Anger

Anger is a common response children have as a result of changes in their lives. Although it may not be a parent's first response, anger should be thought of as a gift the child presents to the parents. A child's anger is usually open and direct, so it is easier to address. Anger can be directed at the ill parent, the healthy parent, the child's teacher, friends, or God. Anger becomes more troublesome when it is directed inward. It builds up if kept inside. Exploring the anger with your child, offering healthy ways of expressing it, and providing acceptance of it can be your gift back to your child.

Guilt

Children often think they caused their parent's illness. They may blame themselves for things that go wrong. They question what they did to cause the illness. They may think if they are "very, very good" their parent will get better—as a direct result of their behavior. Children also sometimes feel guilty because they are well, and their parent is sick. They may feel it's not right for them to enjoy things they like to do when the person with cancer can't do what he or she likes.

Physical Symptoms

Sometimes it's hard for children to express emotional pain verbally, so they may express it physically through a variety of ailments or injuries. By drawing attention to physical discomfort, children command the attention that they might not get otherwise. This can be handled in an understanding, but not overly responsive manner. It is best to divert attention away from their physical complaints and focus your attention on positive behaviors. For some children, it may be necessary to discuss this way of coping and discourage its use. Assuring a child that he or she has your attention without being ill may be all that is needed.

Sleep Problems

Children also cannot divert themselves from their troubles when they need to rest and sleep. Therefore, some children will have a hard time letting go at night and falling asleep. Others may fall asleep and awaken early. Some will sleep too much in order to avoid reality. Teens are famous for oversleeping. Nightmares may happen because children are not able to directly express their feelings and concerns.

Regression

All parents delight in their children's growth and healthy development. So, it is upsetting to observe children regressing, or going backward, in their development. Temper tantrums, long ago tamed, may suddenly become a problem. Children, who had improved their tendency to whine, may suddenly whine more. Teens, who enjoyed an active social life, may begin to withdraw and demand more parental attention. All of these are examples of regression. Usually these things are short-lived and will come to pass.

Eating Problems

Changes in eating habits are a sign of distress in children. Food may become an area where children can express their frustration with unwanted change and need for control. Children who are picky eaters may become even more discerning. Teens who tend to eat mostly junk food may double their food intake or not eat much at all.

Children's Responses and Their Developmental Levels

Children grow and develop in certain expected ways. Although parents do not need to be child development experts, some information about each developmental stage is critical to understanding and talking with children about cancer. Thinking about the developmental tasks confronting each age group can be helpful when looking at how a cancer diagnosis impacts the children in a family.

Newborns and Infants

John Bowlby was a well-known researcher who studied infants and their attachments to their parents. He concluded that infants as young as six months old could experience grief when separated from a parent. When a parent is ill with cancer, a baby may sense the anxiety in a stressed-out parent's arms or that the parent is not quite as attentive. But in general, most babies are not able to understand illness. This can make it easier for others to take care of their needs when parents cannot. Most people who work with babies would agree that the most important aspect of parenting is a consistent, loving presence, where the babies' needs for nurturing, physical comfort, security, food, and stimulation are met as soon as possible. Infants need regular contact with nurturing caretakers.

Toddlers (1–3 years)

Toddlers are at a stage where they begin to develop a sense of independence and mastery over their environment. They realize that their behavior impacts others. They understand that they are separate entities from their parents. Toddlers are also learning that an object exists even when they cannot see it. They are beginning to use words to interact with others, although what they see is still more important than what they are told. Their thinking centers around themselves and they do not think in a logical pattern.

Toddlers exhibit temper tantrums as a means of expressing their frustration. Their favorite word is "No." Toddlers can tolerate being separated from their parents for brief periods, but are often fearful when strangers are present. Loud noises, sleep, and animals may be other things they fear. When they play with other children, they play beside others, not really with others.

Preschoolers (3–5 years)

As any parent of a preschooler knows, preschoolers are energetic and physically oriented. They play hard and socialize more with friends. They have active imaginations, and tend to think magically. They believe that thinking about something can make it happen. Until about the age of six, they are still figuring out the difference between what is real and what is imagined. They often pretend and play with objects as if they are alive.

Children at this age become upset and frightened by being away from their parents for a long period of time. Many of their fears are about being separated from parents or caretakers. They can find support in security objects, such as a favorite cuddly animal, and can often begin to state their feelings. At this age, children are beginning to learn to use simple words for expressing emotions.

School-Age Children (6–12 years)

Children at this stage are becoming very good with talking and physical skills. They can think about something even if they have not experienced it directly. They understand the concept of something being reversible. This is a time when they begin to seek more independence from their parents. Feedback from their peer group is important to them as they are learning about their own special interests and aptitudes. They have a strong need to feel competent in some unique area.

School-age children have fears about losing control and competence. They fear being alone and not being like their peers. Their relationships with their parents during this period are still very significant, but their network has expanded to include teachers, peers, and other adults.

Teenagers (13–18 years)

The teen years are often called a storm. With some teenagers, this is well deserved! Teens are searching for their own identities, separate from their parents. But, they also fear losing control and independence. While they are pulling away from their parents, they are also pulling in when they need extra support because independence itself can be frightening. They often exhibit mood swings and irrational behavior as their self-esteem ebbs and flows.

This is a time when their bodies are changing rapidly, and they are having sexual thoughts and feelings. They are capable of abstract thinking, logical reasoning, and problem solving. They form their own personal value system at this time, which is often idealistic.

Teens can be painfully self-conscious—and think others are analyzing them constantly. Therefore, privacy is crucial. Their peer group is the most influential force in their lives. They fear being rejected or different from their peers.

About This Book

The information included in this book is based on scientific information combined with many years of clinical experience. In order to enhance our knowledge, we conducted a national survey of group leaders who work with children whose parents have cancer to get their ideas about what has helped them deal with cancer in the family. We spoke with these professionals to get their insights and strategies about what they have seen that helps children adapt, cope, and even thrive. We collected and developed many helpful activities, suggestions, and exercises. You can use the hands-on tools at the end of Chapters 1, 2, 5, and 6 to help your children express their feelings and cope with the emotional effects of cancer in the family.

Book Organization

Chapter 1 explores parents' personal reactions to a diagnosis of cancer and how children typically respond. This chapter contains suggestions for telling children about a cancer diagnosis and how to manage their reactions. It also provides answers to questions commonly asked by children.

Chapter 2 provides suggestions for helping children understand treatment. The specific side effects of treatment and its impact on both parents and children are examined. Often during treatment, separation of some type is required due to hospitalization or relatives taking care of the children. Staying connected during treatment is key and we discuss how to do that in specific ways. This chapter also includes ideas about how to manage discipline at a time when most parents feel depleted.

Chapter 3 explains what psychosocial support services are, how to use them, and where to find them. It offers ways to help you work through the barriers that keep people from getting help. Information about choosing a counselor and paying for services is also included.

Chapter 4 talks about how to take care of yourself, which ultimately helps you take care of your children. This chapter includes suggestions for exercises and techniques to help improve the quality of your life. You can also use many of the exercises along with your children.

Chapter 5 addresses the time after treatment, the "quiet" period that can be surprisingly more emotionally difficult than any other time. It highlights what to expect after treatment and how you and your children can thrive now that treatment is over.

Chapter 6 looks at how families deal with recurrence. Whether recurrence actually occurs or not, it is a concern for most people with cancer. Here, the potential of death is openly addressed and discussed.

Chapter 7 highlights special issues that impact children within the context of a cancer illness. These include single parent and non-traditional households; parents with problems of drug or alcohol abuse; or homes with financial or marital instability. Other losses, such as loss of a peer, friend, teacher, or other relative are explored. AIDS-related cancer also creates special coping issues for children.

KIDS' CORNER. This special removable workbook is filled with exercises your children can use on their own to work through their experiences. This is a place they can use to keep track of their own thoughts and feelings. Many of these exercises can work for your teenagers too if they let themselves be open and creative with the process. This removable booklet is designed especially for children to record their own personal thoughts and feelings, much like a diary. We encourage you to respect their privacy, although they may choose to share some of the material with you.

✑

Children are very observant about things that are happening around them. For example, when ten-year-old Jamie's parents met with a counselor, they told the counselor that their children did not know anything. However, Jamie had seen the sign on the building, "Cancer Center," and suspected her mother had cancer. She also had overheard her father talking earlier about a wig. She understood what that meant because she knew that cancer treatment causes people to lose hair. When leaving the session, Jamie asked, "Why didn't you tell me you had cancer?"

✑

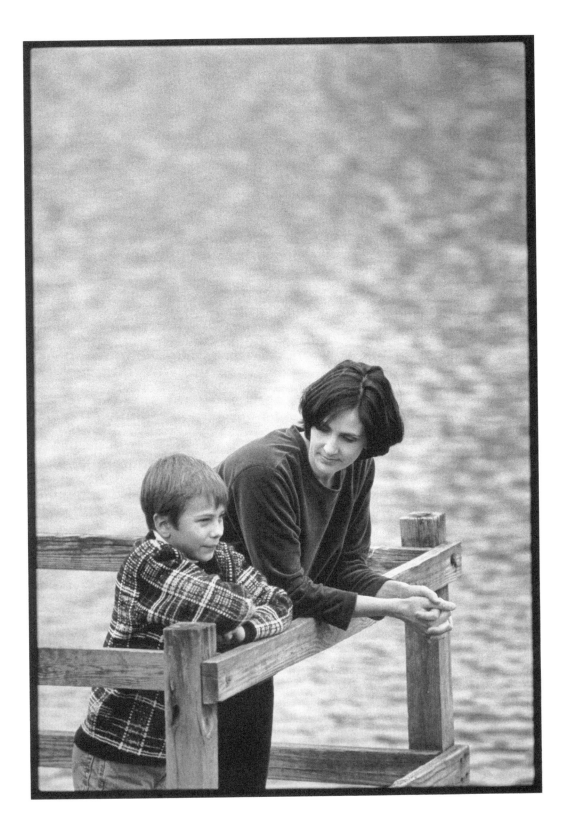

CHAPTER ONE

Helping Children
understand diagnosis

"You have cancer"... "The cells are malignant." No matter how this information is presented, lives are changed the moment cancer is diagnosed. Regardless of the hopeful picture presented with a cancer diagnosis, there is tremendous fear, shock, and dread associated with this diagnosis. Still today, people think of death, suffering, and isolation.

In addition to experiencing all the usual reactions, parents' responses are also intensified by thinking of cancer's impact on their children. Parents never want their children to feel pain or suffer insecurity. A cancer diagnosis brings all those worries to the surface, even if the outlook is good.

There are many things that impact how someone responds to a cancer diagnosis, such as the losses someone has suffered in the past, how the person reacted to that loss, what type of support system is in place, and a person's spiritual beliefs, values, and culture. Those same factors also impact a child's response.

Parents can benefit from discussing with a significant other, minister, or good friend how they are feeling emotionally about the diagnosis. This can help them prepare for talking with their children. Practicing potential reactions with others may help diminish some painful aspects of sharing the news with children.

Opening the Door to Communication

You may feel alone and as though you are the only one affected by your cancer. But your partner, your children, and your friends are also struggling with the complex emotions involved with cancer. Cancer affects the entire family. Each person in your family has to deal with your cancer in his or her own way. Some family members may want to take charge of organizing help for you in order to feel more in control. Other family members may want to avoid the situation and pretend it is not happening. Talk to your family and get everyone to share their feelings so that fears and concerns can be addressed. The different stresses that cancer brings can challenge even the best functioning families. But, depending on how everyone responds, cancer can also bring people closer and provide a deeper appreciation of each other.

Finding a way to talk to your children about your illness and how it's likely to impact the family is an important part of helping them cope. You can use the activities at the end of this chapter as tools for communication. Communication can be difficult, even if the family has done well discussing issues in the past, because cancer and its treatment brings up feelings that can be hard to talk about. Sometimes people use silence as a way to protect themselves or each other from fear, upsetting thoughts, or feelings. But, withholding or denying real feelings eventually leads to more problems.

You should not keep a cancer diagnosis secret. It is better to talk with children about what is happening. Some parents think that their children will worry more if they are told the facts about the situation. But, research shows that talking about a parent's cancer diagnosis helps lower children's anxiety and improves family communications in general. Children also have not had the same life experiences as adults and usually do not respond the same emotionally to cancer. Trying to protect children by hiding the diagnosis is not a good strategy. Cancer is an impossible secret to keep, and your children will most likely suspect that something is wrong anyway. Even very small children will know that something is terribly wrong. Children can often pick up on the anxiety and worry of their parents. Usually, they fear and believe the worst if they aren't given an honest explanation, and will draw their own conclusions. Children can feel rejected if their parents are being secretive and conclude that they don't love them anymore or are being punished for being "bad." In addition, the effort it takes to keep such a secret may rob you of precious energy.

Trying to keep a cancer diagnosis secret can also cause children to feel that whatever is happening is too terrible to talk about. This can create an exaggerated sense of doom. It can also cause children to feel very isolated from the family. So, the natural desire parents have to protect their children usually backfires and only makes things harder. Parents know that it is impossible to shield children from all of the stressful parts of life, and that their job is to teach their children how to cope with these challenges.

You are a role model. How children react to a cancer diagnosis depends a great deal on how their parents or other close adults are handling the crisis. Children understand through their parents what is happening in their world. While parents know this, it can be very stressful, because they will be dealing with their own powerful feelings of fear and uncertainty. However, parents and their children can and do learn to cope with cancer and its treatments. One survivor said, "I wish I would have been more open with my children instead of trying to shield and protect them. I think I could have prevented some of the acting out behaviors that I saw. I think they needed to be more involved to help both themselves and me."

What Other Children May Say

When a five-year-old boy told a friend at school that his mother had cancer, the classmate gave a very frightening response. He said his mother had cancer and she died, so the boy's mother was also going to die. The boy then asked his mother every day when she was going to die. Because the mother's cancer was diagnosed at a very early stage, she told her son that her cancer was very treatable. She explained that while some people die from cancer, many other people survive. "Your friend's mom is different from me. I am taking medicine that will make me get better," she said, "I am lucky because they found it early and I can get the help I need." Eventually he stopped asking this question every day when she continued to reassure him that what happened to his friend's mother would not be likely to happen to her.

You are the best source of information. Children should be given information by their parents. If children hear about their parent's cancer from someone else such as a curious neighbor or a classmate who has heard other people talking, it can harm the trust that should exist between parents and their children. If children think their parents are being vague or are trying to hide something from them, they will have difficulty believing they are being told the truth. The parent must do everything possible to maintain trust. So it is better that parents learn how to communicate this information truthfully, but in a way that allows children to understand and participate in what is happening in their lives.

Be as honest and sensitive as you can. It will help children adjust to this difficult situation and may influence the way in which they deal with change in the future if you are straightforward. Answer whatever questions children have as openly and clearly as you can, and allow them to react emotionally to what's happening. This way you will teach children how to cope with the challenges of cancer as well as they can. This is a time of learning for both you and your children.

Try not to hide your feelings. If you never show your feelings, chances are your children won't either. Covering up strong emotions is like sitting on a time bomb. Eventually the feelings will explode. Parents can lead by example by admitting fear. You can explain, "It is a really scary time right now, but we know that it won't always feel like this." If you are honest with your feelings, they will know it's okay to share their own. If you try to hide your feelings, your children can become frightened of their own feelings instead of accepting them.

The first discussion should not be your last. Keep in mind that communicating with children about cancer is not a one-time event. It is a process that will continue over time. As treatment progresses, new issues and concerns will arise. Keep children posted throughout the illness. If the illness goes into an extended remission or continues as a chronic problem, children will need updates tailored to their own changing understanding and emotional needs.

Talking with Your Children

Timing Is Everything

The discussion with children about a cancer diagnosis should come before the treatment begins and at a point when the parents can discuss it openly and calmly. Not too much time should elapse after learning about the diagnosis. It should take place in the home, in a quiet atmosphere where no one needs to rush off to keep another appointment. There needs to be plenty of time for questions and expressing feelings.

It is best to have the nuclear family involved in the discussion; family members should be told before outsiders. Naturally, if an outside person or relative is close to the children, it may be important to involve them as well. In a two-parent household, it is advisable for parents to talk to their children together. It helps to have the person affected by the cancer explain what is happening. This reassures the children that they are able to talk about it and that the children have permission to talk about it in the future. For single parents, it may be a good idea to ask a relative or friend to be with them if they're feeling a bit shaky about the conversation.

It is good for parents to choose a time when they are feeling fairly calm to talk to their children. If you are feeling distraught or uncertain about what to say, it might be better to wait until your emotions are a bit more under control.

Communication Tips

- Timing is important. Make sure you choose a time that will be uninterrupted and does not take place before a major school or extracurricular event.
- Emphasize the process over the content. How you say something is more important than what you say.
- Answer the specific question that is asked. Providing more information than requested can be overwhelming.
- Make sure your explanations are appropriate for the child's age.

That is not to say that you need to pretend that there is nothing to worry about, or that it's terrible if your children see you crying. You can acknowledge that this is an upsetting time, that cancer is a scary disease, and that it's okay to have strong feelings about it. But, that doesn't mean that the family won't be able to find ways to cope.

Obviously, what people tell their children depends a great deal on how they understand their particular cancer and its prognosis. Even with a very uncertain future, parents will still need to focus on what they have to do to live with their illness. Children will need to do the same. Regardless of the words that are used, one of the most important things for parents to communicate is their willingness to tell the truth. This does not mean that parents should tell their children all that they know as soon as they know it. It means that children should be given truthful information, when they need to have it, to cope with what is happening to them. For example, a good way to say this is, "I don't want you to worry about the future at this point. Let's think about what's going on right now. If that should change, I promise you I will tell you. I will always try to tell you the truth. I want you to ask me any questions you have and I'll do my best to answer them." The goal is to give children a balanced point of view. They should realize that cancer is a serious but not a hopeless illness.

Consider Your Child's Developmental Stage

A child's age is an important factor in deciding what and how much you should tell about a new diagnosis. For example, an adolescent daughter of a woman with breast cancer will have different concerns than a six-year-old girl who needs a parent for basic caregiving. The guiding principle should be to tell the truth in such a way that the child is able to understand and prepare for the changes that will happen in the family. You may want to ask a social worker, school counselor, or other parents in your position how they have explained cancer to children that are your youngsters' ages.

When talking to children, use simple, age-appropriate language based on what is really happening. All children need the following basic information: the name of the cancer, such as "breast cancer," or "lymphoma," the part of the body where the cancer is, how it will be treated, and how their own lives will be affected. Although they may not respond right away, be prepared to answer whatever questions may come up and allow them to show their emotions.

They may react more to how you are behaving than to what you are saying. It's also okay to tell them that you do not have all the answers.

Talking with Newborns, Infants, and Toddlers

Obviously it is not necessary to talk with infants about the diagnosis. Infants and babies up to age two are too young to understand an illness such as cancer. They can't see it or touch it and are more concerned with what's happening to them. Being separated from parents is a major worry at this stage. Children more than a year old are concerned with how things feel and how to control things around them. You can describe the illness to toddlers in the simplest possible terms. For example, "Mommy has a boo-boo. Mommy's medicine makes her hair go away, but Mommy will be okay."

Talking with Preschoolers

Preschoolers are better able to understand illness, although they will not need a great deal of detailed information. Begin by asking what they understand or think about the illness. Using simple explanations with dolls or pictures can help. For example, the father could draw a picture of himself with a circle in his stomach where the cancer is located. Preschoolers tend to focus on the visible symptoms of illness rather than the abstract concept of cancer. Demonstrating on a doll or stuffed animal may also make this more concrete. Younger preschoolers often do not ask questions because they don't know what to ask.

Calm Advice

"Telling your children is the hardest part. It is essential that you think through what you're going to say as the words and emotions will have a significant impact on how the children will react. The calmer you are, the less frightened they will be…. As calm as we were, the revelation of cancer was a huge shock to our kids and was met with fear and tears. It is essential that kids are reassured that their parents are going to do everything possible in the way of treatment, that they are still deeply loved and always will be, and if necessary, assured none of this is their fault."

Therefore, simple but full explanations are recommended to anticipate potential questions.

In addition to the illness itself, there are other worries children have
about cancer. The most common of these is that something they did or didn't
do may have caused the parent's illness. While we know this isn't true, most
children believe this at some point during the experience. Preschoolers engage
in "magical thinking," which means they think the world revolves around
them and they believe they can make all kinds of things happen. So, they need
to understand that they are not responsible for the illness.

Because young children are afraid of separation, strangers, and being
alone, they need reassurance that they will not be abandoned. Let them know
that there will always be someone who will take care of them. Assure them
that you're doing everything possible to get better. Explain that there may be
times your mind is on other things, but that doesn't mean you have forgotten
about them. They also tend to get upset if they see prolonged expressions of
sadness by their parents. So, even though a little bit of expressed sadness is
okay by the parents, it should be kept to a minimum.

Talking with School-Age Children

Older children (e.g., ages six to twelve) may be able to understand a more
complex explanation of the cancer diagnosis. At this point, children may have
been taught about cells of the body. They may be interested in seeing pictures
of cancer cells or learning more about it from their parents. Cancer cells can
be described as cells that grow that don't belong there. All the cells form
together in a ball, which is called a tumor. Treatment will involve taking medicine to kill the cells or having a surgeon take it out. School-age children may
particularly benefit from books with stories and descriptions of cancer-related
experiences.

School-age children can also believe that bad things happen because
they have been angry with their parents or because they were naughty. So
when a parent gets sick, children often feel guilty and think they are to blame
for the cancer. Kids usually won't express this, so it's a good idea to reassure
them. It is important to let children know that your illness is not their fault
and that no one can cause someone else to get cancer. It's better not to wait to
see if children bring this up because it may not happen for a long time and in
the meantime, they may feel guilty for no reason.

Reassurance about how they will be cared for is very important. They need to know how their routines will be maintained or how they will change. Consistency in their care is key. Children at this stage can handle some emotional expression by their parents, but this needs to be controlled and modeled for them. They also need reassurance that the well parent will not develop cancer.

Older school-age children need to know the name of the illness, its progress, symptoms, treatments, and potential causes. They need to know the relationship between the illness and the behavior and appearance of the parent. They also need to know what the outcome of the illness will be. They may be able to reverse some of the magical thinking process described earlier. At this stage, they can logically tell themselves that the cancer is not their fault, with reinforcement from parents.

Talking with Teenagers

Teenagers are able to understand complex relationships between events. They are able to think about things they have not experienced themselves. They may define the illness by specific symptoms, such as fatigue, but they are able to understand the reasons for the symptoms. They should have as much information about your diagnosis as they seem prepared to hear and you feel they need to know.

The teen years are a time when children are learning to become independent from the family, so their concerns about you and the new responsibilities going on at home conflict with their need to separate. They may be angry and rebellious. The need for continued independence should be openly addressed. Encourage them to talk about their feelings with you and other people they trust. It may be embarrassing for a young male to talk about his mother having breast cancer, so having others to talk to can be helpful.

The reality of having to deal with a cancer diagnosis in and of itself sets teenagers apart from their peers. They are "different" as a result. Because conformity is so important, this can be a curse to a teenager. Their peers may be agonizing over who is going to the weekend party, while they are worried about having a parent live. The differences are striking.

A Story is Worth a Thousand Words

One way to think about cancer and what it means is to compare it to a garden. Gardens grow herbs, flowers, and vegetables. But, weeds also grow in a garden and may keep the good plants from growing. Cancer cells in a person's body are like the weeds in the garden. They can harm the good cells and keep them from growing. When weeds come up in a garden, they are pulled out, dug up, and removed in some way. Cancer cells must also be removed from the body. We may use surgery to take the cells out or other ways to kill the cancer cells. These ways are called chemotherapy (use phonetics here) or radiation therapy. These treatments help rid the body of the cancer cells, just like chopping out the weeds helps get them out of the garden.

ഉറ

Children's Common Questions

Parents often avoid conversations about cancer with their children because they're afraid of answering difficult questions. However, thinking about potential questions and responses will help you be prepared. The answers to all questions should be honest, but as optimistic as the situation allows. For example, "This is a serious illness, but I am getting the best possible treatment and the doctor thinks I am responding very well." When optimism is not realistic, parents need to acknowledge how difficult it is to live with uncertainty and to emphasize their determination to confront whatever happens together as a family. While these questions may not be asked directly, we know from experience with other families that these are questions children think about when a parent gets cancer. While you will not know the answers to all of these questions, especially when you are first diagnosed, these are issues that need to be discussed at some point in your experience.

"Are You Going to Die?"

This is the question that all parents dread. The question about the possibility of death is the one that causes the most distress to families. Some children may not ask about it up front, but this is the worry that is on everyone's mind within the family.

By around the age of eight, children can begin to understand death as a permanent state. It is a good idea to rehearse how you are going to respond to this either with someone else or in your own head. There are some things you should know before you decide how to answer this question. The first is that this is a very scary question for children to ask and they may never have the courage to ask it directly. It does, however, need to be addressed, as it will be something that will probably worry them.

Another point is that there is usually no way to tell for sure at the beginning of the cancer experience if a person will die. The answer to the question depends on the patient's response to treatment. Even for cancers with a very poor outlook, a person's response to treatment is the key to how they will do. Cancer is a chronic disease, not necessarily a terminal one.

If you expect the person with cancer to make a full recovery with treatment, you can certainly state that. If things are more serious, it is appropriate to say something like, "It is going to be a tough fight, but I am getting treatment and I should respond to it. I will let you know how it's going every step of the way."

Even people with serious cancers can live for many years. You will need to set the stage that you and the family will be living with cancer. Focusing the family on how to live with cancer, not how to die with it can be a constructive interpretation of events. For cancers that are metastatic or have spread to other parts of the body at diagnosis, parents will need to be more direct and give children different information (see Chapter 6).

What You Can Say

Here are some examples of what other parents have said in response to this question:

- Sometimes people do die from cancer; I'm not expecting that to happen because the doctors have told me they have very good treatments these days.
- Many people are cured of cancer these days, that's why I'm getting treatment.
- The doctors have told me that my chances of being cured are very good. I think we should believe them until they tell us otherwise. I'll let you know if that changes.
- There is no way to know right now what's going to happen until I get some treatment. I think we should feel positive about things for now and hopefully we will feel even better in the future.
- Years ago, people often died from cancer because treatments weren't as good. Now there are a lot more choices of treatment, and the outlook for many cancers is much more hopeful.
- They don't know a lot about the kind of cancer I have. But, I'm certainly going to give it my best.
- My cancer is a tough one to treat, but I'm going to work hard at getting better. We just don't know what is going to happen. The most important thing is that we stick together as a family and let each other know what's going on with all of us. If you can't stop worrying, I want you to tell me because there are things we can do to feel better.
- I don't think I'm going to die. None of us knows for sure. But, I'm going to do everything I can to make sure that doesn't happen.

❧

"Can I or Someone Else Catch It?"

Children often worry that cancer is contagious, or that they or the other parent will get it. It's a good idea to correct these ideas before the children have a chance to worry. Children know they can "catch" a cold by being near someone who is sick, so it makes sense for them to become confused and worry that cancer can be passed from one person to another. Parents can explain that cancer is a different kind of illness and the child doesn't have to worry that someone passed it on to Mom or Dad or that they will get it. Parents should also say that it would be very unusual for the other parent to get sick.

"Is It Inherited?"

Many people believe that cancer typically runs in families. They think that if one family member has it, others will too. But, most people with cancer do not have a form of inherited cancer, nor will they pass it on to their children. Just because someone in the family has cancer doesn't mean that someone else in the family will develop cancer. About 5 percent of people with cancer today will have a form of inherited cancer. People whose close blood relatives have breast cancer, colon cancer, prostate cancer, ovarian cancer, melanoma, Wilms' tumor, or retinoblastoma may be at a slight increased risk for those cancers.

"Did I Cause It?"

The most universal issue for children concerns whose fault it is that Mom or Dad got cancer. It is well known that children blame themselves when something goes wrong. This is common in children of divorcing parents. They often assume it was something they did to cause the breakup of their parents' marriage. The same thing happens with illness—children wonder if they are to blame. As discussed earlier, children may worry that they did or didn't do something to cause their parent's illness. It is best to confront this directly by saying something like, "Nothing any of you did caused the cancer. None of us had anything to do with causing it."

"Is It Going to Hurt?"

Pain is one of the reasons people still fear cancer so much. Having cancer does not necessarily mean you will have pain. Much progress has been made in pain control. Some cancers cause no physical pain at all. Even people with advanced cancers do not always have pain. But, if pain does occur, there are many ways to relieve or reduce it. You can let your children know that there are things that can be done to help relieve your pain. A combination of pain control methods can be used. In addition to surgery and medicines, there are other techniques to help manage pain such as imagery, biofeedback, relaxation, and distraction (see Chapter 4).

Some people are reluctant to take medicines for pain because they are afraid they will become addicted. Research has shown that people with cancer can take pain medicines as long as needed, if used properly, without becoming addicted. People also worry that if they take their medicines continuously, they will become "immune" to that dosage and need higher doses until no dosage will work. In reality, increasing the dosage for most prescribed medicines increases their effectiveness.

"Is Cancer a Punishment?"

Children sometimes have mistaken ideas about punishment, guilt, and how to fix things. Some children worry that if they misbehave, they may be punished with a disease. It's important to let them know that people don't get sick because of what they did or did not do in the past. Cancer does not discriminate between "good" people and "bad" people. The disease cuts across all lines including race, religion, and gender.

"Does Radiation Treatment Make People Radioactive?"

Radiation treatments are painless, like having an x-ray picture taken, and do not cause people to become radioactive. You can let your children know that they won't become radioactive by touching you. External radiation therapy affects targeted cells only for a moment. With internal radiation therapy, the radiation is placed inside you and your body may emit a small amount of radiation for only a short time. If the internal radiation is contained in a closed implant, the radioactive material cannot escape. To ensure visitors' protection, precautions are taken anyway and may include hospitalization and limitation of visitors. You can tell your children that it is safe to touch you and that your body does not contain enough radioactivity to be dangerous to others.

"What Is Going to Happen to Me?"

The bottom line for most children is what is going to happen to them. Many children wonder who will take care of their needs when a parent is sick. Not only might children fear the loss of the ill parent, but they can also easily transfer that fear of loss to the remaining healthy parent or other caregiver. When one bad thing happens in the family, children sense that bad things can happen that are out of their control.

Children need to know how their routines will be affected and who is going to do the things you have been doing for them. When changes in the routine are necessary, these should be done with the assurance that the changes are temporary. Explain in detail who will be responsible for maintaining particular activities such as cooking, taking children to various activities, and so on. It is helpful to explain to children how chores will be divided and roles will be changing. Discuss what will happen, when it will happen, and who will be involved.

Children's Reactions to the News About Diagnosis

Children of all ages are affected by a parent's cancer diagnosis. Children's emotional reactions to this news depend on many things, including how the information is presented, their past experiences with pain and illness, and their age.

Reactions Based on Age

Newborns and Infants

Babies may be fussier during this time. They will notice the lack of consistent caregivers and cry from separation anxiety. Their needs may not be met as quickly or in the same way. They may also sense the general unrest of the household, which will be reflected in their eating and sleeping behaviors.

Toddlers

Toddlers are also affected by the separations that will occur as a result of a new diagnosis of cancer in the family. They don't understand what cancer is, but they understand changes in family routines and how they impact their lives directly. As part of normal development, toddlers often express negativity. This may be exaggerated in the family experiencing stress, and it may progress into tantrums or withdrawal. Toddlers are unable to empathize with or understand what is going on. However, with effort made toward maintaining routines and keeping them interested and diverted, this can be avoided. If some progression in toilet training is slowed due to the circumstances, understand they will resume this activity when they feel ready.

Preschoolers

Preschoolers have the capacity to understand a little bit more deeply than toddlers about the physical process that is occurring with cancer. Again, however, their response will be egocentric (self-centered). They focus on how the cancer will affect them. In the beginning, it may not have much impact on them. Once separations begin, there will be a more noticeable effect.

Preschoolers express their distress and frustration by yelling, refusing to cooperate, and even destroying objects. It is difficult for them to actually "talk" about their feelings. However, they may benefit a great deal from having the opportunity to talk. Parents can paraphrase for them what their behavior might mean. For example, "It seems like it really makes you mad when we talk about Mommy's cancer. Do you feel sad too?" Preschoolers also express their feelings through play. Careful observation of play may provide valuable information about their adjustment.

School-Age Children

School-age children may act sad and dejected by the news of a cancer diagnosis. They may also act angry, irritable, and disappointed. They may personalize their parent's illness, meaning they interpret parental behavior as responses to their own bad behavior. Still, children this age need their parents for nurturing, security, and support.

The degree that the illness prevents school-aged children from interacting with their peers is significant, since these relationships are becoming very important. They may feel a lack of competence, which can also lead to even more frustration and regression.

Teenagers

The detailed information that parents may give teens about the illness can cause fairly strong emotional reactions. However, many teens try to control these reactions, which can lead to withdrawal and an even more pronounced need for privacy. Other teens express their anger strongly, along with feelings of depression and anxiety.

The news that there is cancer in the family can reinforce the feelings of separateness from their peers, which is often painful for teenagers. On the other hand, teenagers want to be and act grown up. So, sometimes they fall prey to acting over-responsible and not allowing themselves to be teenagers.

What You Can Do

How you and your children respond to a diagnosis of cancer depends a great deal on their age. The following chart on the next two pages describes children's understanding about illness and examples of how they may react at different stages. Some suggestions about how you can manage the situation are provided. These are general guidelines, so you will need to determine what is most likely to apply for each of your children. Some of the suggestions for one age group may also work for a different age group, depending on the development of each child.

Expressing Feelings

Sometimes parents worry about expressing any negative emotions in front of their children. They worry that this will frighten the children or that their "negativity" will somehow impact their ability to get better. Obviously, no one wants to alarm their children by being hysterical. However, there is absolutely nothing wrong with shedding a few tears when a crisis happens in a family. Parents can tell their children that there will be times when they will need to cry about the situation as that helps them to feel better. Parents can assure them that "everyone always stops crying" and that crying does not mean that the situation is worse. It models a way to handle feelings and gives children permission to express their very normal angry and scared feelings. Sharing emotions can also strengthen the bond between parents and children. Everyone deals with problems in a different way and it will be important for parents to give themselves permission and time to figure out what is best for them and their families.

In families in which many people have died of cancer, children may assume the worst possible outcome. So it is important for parents to explain that there are over one hundred different kinds of cancer, that they are all different in their biology, the kind of treatment they need, what is likely to happen in the future, and so on. Make sure they understand that each situation is unique and that just because Grandpa died five years ago doesn't mean that will happen now. Everyone responds differently to treatment and cancer treatment changes from year to year as more effective treatments are being developed all the time. No one can predict the future and people deserve to approach cancer treatment with as much hope as possible.

AGE GROUP	CHILDREN'S UNDERSTANDING OF ILLNESS	CHILDREN'S POSSIBLE REACTIONS	PARENT'S POSSIBLE RESPONSES
Newborns/ Infants/Toddlers	• They have little awareness of illness. • Infants are aware of feelings parents show including anxiety. • They are aware of periods of separation from parents. • They can get upset when the presence of a physical and loving parent is missing. • Toddlers may react to physical changes in parent or presence of side effects (e.g., vomiting).	• fussy and cranky • crying • clinging • change in sleeping or eating habits • colic • slight skin rash • toddlers: tantrums, more negativity • returns to thumb sucking, bedwetting, baby talk, etc.	• Provide consistent caretaking by maintaining baby's schedule. • Ask family members and friends to help with household tasks and care. • Give plenty of physical contact (patting, hugging, holding). • Observe play for clues to their adjustment. • Provide daily contact to help them feel secure. • Express your feelings and fears with others. • Use relaxation tapes, music, or baby massage.
Preschoolers (3–5 years)	• They have a beginning level of understanding about illness. • Children may believe that they caused the illness (e.g., by being angry with parents, thinking bad thoughts). This is an example of magical thinking. • Children consider themselves the center of the universe. They are egocentric and think everything is related to them. • Children may think they can catch the same thing. • Illness may be seen as punishment for being bad.	• thumb sucking • fear of the dark, monsters, animals, darkness, strangers, and the unknown • nightmares • sleepwalking, sleeptalking • bedwetting • stuttering • baby talk • hyperactivity • apathy • fear of separation from significant others (especially at bedtime or going to preschool) • aggression (e.g., hitting, biting)	• Talk about the illness with pictures, dolls, or stuffed animals. Read a picture book about the illness. • Read a story about nightmares or other problems (e.g., *There's A Nightmare in My Closet*). • Explain what they can expect; describe how things may change regarding routines, activities, and schedules. • Reassure them that they will be taken care of and will not be forgotten. • Provide brief and simple explanations. Repeat explanations when necessary. • Encourage them to have fun. • Show emotion with some caution. • Assure them that they have not caused the illness by their behavior or thoughts. • Paraphrase for children what their behavior might mean. • Continue usual discipline and limit setting. Provide outlets for aggression that are positive (see Chapter 2). • Be sure children get physical activity to use up excess energy and anxiety. • Assure them they cannot catch the illness.

AGE GROUP	CHILDREN'S UNDERSTANDING OF ILLNESS	CHILDREN'S POSSIBLE REACTIONS	PARENT'S POSSIBLE RESPONSES
School Age Children (6–12 years)	• They are able to understand more complex explanations of cancer diagnosis. Can understand what cancer cells are. • They still may feel responsible for causing illness because of bad behavior. • Nine years old and older understand that parent can die.	• irritable • sad, crying • anxiety, guilt, jealousy • physical complaints: headaches, stomachaches • separation anxiety at time of going to school or away to camp • hostile reactions toward sick parent, like yelling or fighting • poor concentration, daydreaming, lack of attention • poor grades • withdrawal • difficulty adapting to change • fear of performance, punishment, or new situations • sensitivity to shame and embarrassment	• Use books to explain illness, treatment, and potential outcome (e.g., *Our Mom Has Cancer*). • Assure them that they did not cause the illness by their behaviors or thoughts. • Reassure them about their care and schedule. • Tell them the other parent is healthy. • Let them know how they can help. • Take time to listen and let them know you care about their feelings. • Address issue of parent dying even if children do not bring up topic. • See Chapter 2 for ways to help children express feelings and deal with stress. • See also suggestions for preschool age children.
Teenagers (13–18 years)	• They are capable of abstract thinking; can think about things they have not experienced themselves. • Able to begin thinking more like adults. • Able to understand that people are fragile. • Able to understand complex relationships between events. • Able to understand reasons for symptoms. • More likely to deny fear and worry in order to avoid discussion.	• want to be more independent and treated like adults • anger and rebellion • may criticize how parents handle illness situation • depression • anxiety • worry about being different • poor judgment • withdrawal • apathy • physical symptoms: stomachaches, headaches, rashes • more likely to turn feelings inward (so parents are less likely to see reactions)	• Encourage them to talk about their feelings, but realize they may find it easier to confide in friends, teachers, or other trusted people. • Provide plenty of physical and verbal expressions of love. • Talk about role changes in family. • Provide privacy as needed. • Encourage them to maintain activities and peer relationships. • If problems are noted, provide opportunities for counseling. • Set appropriate limits. • Don't rely on them to take on too many added responsibilities. • Provide resources for learning more about the disease and getting support. • See also suggestions for school-age children.

As mentioned before, children's reactions to the news of a parent's illness depend on many things. The age of the children, their personalities, their relationships to their parents, and the way information is presented are just a few factors that can influence how children will behave. Parents know their children best and can expect that their children will react in ways that are typical of their personalities. For instance, a child who is very dependent may become even more so in the throws of a parent's cancer diagnosis. A child who always imagines the worst may do so now as well. A child who plays rough with toys when upset may get even rougher. Children are often unable to express how they are feeling in words. Most parents get an idea about what is going on with their kids by watching their behavior. So, a parent who is observing their children fighting with each other more now can probably assume that this is their way of showing they're upset. Parents may want to put this into words by saying something like, "I know everybody is more worried right now but let's find a way to talk about this rather than fighting."

Temporary Setbacks

In general, parents can expect that where children are in their overall development will determine their ability to understand what is going on. Children tend to "regress" or go backward when they are under stress. Adults often do the same. A child who has just become toilet trained may start having accidents. A child who has gone off to kindergarten quite happily may become upset at the prospect of separating from a parent. Children, who have been diagnosed with problems in paying attention in school, may have more difficulties for a time. Usually, these behavioral changes disappear after the situation returns to normal.

The other issue that will impact children's behavior at this time is their ability to trust in their parents. Generally, children who are included in this experience from the beginning with truthful information in manageable doses will experience less anxiety than children whose parents are more evasive about what is happening.

Sometimes children react very negatively to changes in routine and parents will feel frustrated and even angry as they try to meet everyone's needs. Keep in mind that it is no one's fault when a parent gets cancer and while there is nothing they can do to change that fact, people do have choices about how to handle the situation. Find something in the situation that the children have a choice about, such as who they would like to have meet the school bus or what they would like to wear when they go to a neighbor's after school. Don't spend endless time negotiating—sometimes that's just the way things have to be at the moment. Children are not expected to like it when their routines are disrupted—adults don't like it either. Parents can acknowledge this to their children along with the fact that they have a right to feel angry and upset right now. Although parents can't change the situation, they will want to know how their children are feeling about all that is going on.

Providing Comfort and Reassurance

A cancer diagnosis may be the first family crisis your children have faced. If they have already experienced loss or serious illness, their previous fears and anxieties will probably affect their coping now. The way parents cope with the emotional and practical disruptions of cancer will set the stage for how the children will deal with them. Children often react more to how parents behave than to what they actually say.

Unfortunately, parents probably cannot offer the kind of reassurance they would like to at the beginning of their experience with cancer. This is because no one really knows at that point how the patient will respond to treatment. In spite of this, there are things that parents can do to help their children begin coping with this new reality. Parents can say that even though they can't see into the future, they can promise that the children will be taken care of. If the parent is feeling sick, they will arrange for someone else to fill in. The most important psychological issue for children is their own sense of security and safety. Children depend on their parents for their basic physical and emotional needs. A parent's cancer diagnosis can make families feel that their lives are totally out of control emotionally.

Children often need frequent reassurance that they'll be safe, secure, and loved. Cancer and its treatment require many absences from home and youngsters are often left in the care of others for periods of time. One of the things children get mad about is feeling left out or neglected. Some feel that they don't get as much attention as before, and they often are right. Parents have a lot on their minds at this time, which may not leave much time for children—

especially if parents are making frequent trips to the clinic or hospital. Children need reassurance that they are not being abandoned and that their parents are always going to make sure they are okay, no matter what happens.

Managing Changing Roles and Daily Routines

Children thrive on routine—it helps them feel safe. When life becomes unpredictable, they need help in adjusting to the changes. During this time, it is important to realize that the entire family is likely to feel anxious and unsettled. You will need to be making trips to the hospital, your partner may be taking time off from work, and the emotions in the household may be strained. You may not be able to do all the things you did before, and you may feel guilty about needing to have others tend to your duties. One survivor said, "Healing is a selfish thing. No one can do it for you. If you're going to be selfish, then be really selfish. We're socialized into taking care of others. We must take care of ourselves."

In spite of this, parents should try to keep as much of their children's lives the same as possible. This may sound like a tall order when the adults are feeling so anxious, but it is possible to reorganize family routines at least temporarily. In talking about your diagnosis and treatment, it is a good idea to prepare children for the fact that certain changes will need to be made in the family routine. Parents will need to call on others for help to fill in for them during periods of active treatment. Perhaps a relative will be moving in temporarily to help out if a parent needs to be hospitalized. Perhaps the parent has friends who have volunteered to take turns in preparing dinners for the family. A relative or friend may volunteer to pick a child up from school and take him to special activities.

Some parents may find it difficult to ask for help. Families may be separated geographically, or there may be a history of family tension. We know from experience that people who try to manage the problems that cancer can cause alone will have a hard time. Try to remember that more often than not, people really do want to help. And, if you allow them to help, they will experience much satisfaction. If there is no one to call on, parents or their families should ask to talk with the hospital social worker or the nurse in the doctor's office because there may be community agencies that can help.

When changes in family routines are explained to children, they offer a powerful message that Mom or Dad is still in charge and the children's needs will be met. Life will go on as normally as possible given the crisis the family is facing and the children will not be left "on their own." Parents should acknowledge that no one is happy that life seems turned upside down right now, but it will be temporary until whatever is going on is completed. Remind them that things won't always be this way. In the meantime, reassure your children that they are loved and that their daily needs will be met. Let them know their daily activities will still continue. They'll still be able to eat their favorite sandwiches for lunch, go to softball practice, play with their friends, and so on.

Whatever needs to be done by way of caregiving will vary depending on the age of your children and availability of other people to help. Obviously, young children may be more of a concern because they have more basic survival needs to be met and are more dependent on the parent. Teenagers can present special challenges because they will be testing out their ability to be independent but can logically be expected to fill in more for an absent or ill parent. It can sometimes be a fine line between asking for help from an adolescent and giving them too much responsibility for the day-to-day running of the household. It may be useful for parents to recognize their teenagers' normal desire for independence and reassure them that you know they will need their own time and

(*continued on page 28*)

Call in the Troops!

Now is the time to work through your own reluctance as a parent and adult to ask for help. No one can manage the cancer experience alone. Your family shouldn't have to either. When a friend or acquaintance states, "If there is anything I can do..." have your list ready. Most people are eager to help someone in this situation. They need the specific suggestions that you have made. If it's difficult to do it for yourself, think of how you are modeling for your children that life is so much more difficult when you do it alone. When one parent or caregiver doesn't feel very emotionally available to their children, chances are that another adult will have just the right touch, just the right way to elicit the feelings you have been unable to.

☙❧

Communicating with Children About Cancer

Being included in the information and education process and feeling that every-one has a role helps family members, especially children, comprehend the physical and emotional challenges of the cancer experience, feel more in con-trol, and provide support where it counts. As with adults, information demystifies cancer and helps children feel more in control. It's important for children of any age to know:

- They did not cause the cancer. It's not their fault you got sick. Cancer is a very complex disease.
- You feel bad because of the illness and treatment, not because of anything they have done.
- Cancer is not contagious, and they don't have to worry about catching it from you.
- Cancer is not a death sentence. More people are cured by today's treatments, and new treatments continue to be developed.
- There are lots of other children whose parents have had cancer. At least 8.4 million Americans alive today have a history of cancer.
- It is normal to have many strong feelings about your illness. People in the family may be upset at times.
- When they get upset, it doesn't mean they are bad people or they don't love the person with cancer. It just means they're upset.
- They can do things to help you and the family work through any changes that are needed.
- They are still allowed to carry on with school, friends, and regular daily activ-ities. It's best for everyone if you give them permission to keep doing things that are important to them.
- It helps to talk about it. Teachers, friends, coaches, neighbors, and extended family members can also provide companionship and support.

Helping Children Cope

- **Talk to your children's teachers.** If parents inform teachers of the family's situation, teachers can be prepared for problems that may occur in school as a result. Even if the outlook for the person with cancer is good, it's important to tell teachers about the situation. Teachers can be an extra source of support and they can also provide information about how the child is coping (see Chapter 2). Children who were having problems at school before the cancer will probably have a worse time now. Intervention before the problems have consequences can save time, money, and stress. Counseling may help them manage their increased distress without experiencing prolonged consequences for their schoolwork and peer relationships.

- **Develop a support network for your children.** Seeing to your children's emotional and physical needs can be extraordinarily difficult in the face of illness-related absences or disability, especially in a single parent household or if the other parent has to work extra hours to compensate for lost earnings or increased costs. You may need to call on friends and relatives to provide childcare.

- **Maintain your children's normal routines.** Allow children to take part in their usual activities in and out of school as much as possible. Routines are important in giving children the security they need to stay on their developmental track. Adolescents in particular need to continue to spend time with their peers and have their privacy.

- **Continue usual discipline with your children.** Children need to know their limits, especially at times of disruption. Discipline problems can arise if children attempt to get the attention they feel they are missing.

- **Involve your children in projects to help.** Give children something to do if they want to be involved, whether it's caring for household pets, helping with meals, or keeping track of timetables. Giving them practical tasks can help them feel useful and more in control of the situation.

- **Ask your children what they think.** Asking for your children's input into resolving some of the home management issues that emerge when dealing with an illness within the family may provide a much-needed sense of competence.

- **Allow your children to have fun without feeling guilty.** Encourage children to keep doing the things they did before you were diagnosed, such as going out with friends, playing games, and joining extracurricular activities.

space in spite of the fact that a parent is ill. Establishing a time for a "family meeting" in which parents and children can review how things are going in the family and make decisions about what should be different or stay the same may also be helpful.

Hands-On Tools

This chapter has given you guidelines on how to explain cancer to your children and how to recognize their normal responses. After you have told them about your diagnosis and treatment, it's important to continue to have ongoing dialogues with them about your illness and its effects.

The following activities are designed to give you and your children some tools that will help them manage feelings about the illness. But, the most important tool you have is your own knowledge about your children and your skill of listening to their feelings. We encourage you and your children to work together on completing these exercises. They are designed to offer a way for you and your children to talk about how the experiences and feelings related to cancer affect your family.

The activities are designed for various ages. Not all of the exercises will be right for your children. Some of them may be above or below your child's learning level, so you can adjust them as needed. You can also use many of the exercises in any of the chapters at any time from diagnosis, through treatment and recovery.

The most valuable part of these activities is for you and your children to have a chance to be together and learn about each other.

This is also a good time to turn to the special **Kids' Corner** removable workbook at the end of this book. You can give this workbook to your children as a way for them to track their own experiences. If they would prefer, you can select exercises to work along with them.

◆   ***Find stories*** about other people who have had cancer and read them with your children.

◆   ***Make up or find a "slogan"*** to help your family throughout this experience. Make banners, mobiles, or buttons using your special phrase for inspiration.

◆   ***Explain what will be happening to you*** by using a doll. You can also use dolls for other members of your family. With younger children, role play. Children often express what they are really feeling in their play.

◆   ***create a "feeling collage"*** with your children. Gather together a stack of old magazines, scissors, and glue. After the collage is completed, talk with your children about what it means to them.

◆   ***Use a kaleidoscope*** to explain to your children how feelings can change and blend together. Explain to them that they will have many feelings as things may change for a while.

◆   ***Use clay, playdough, crayons, or finger-paints*** and have your children show what they think cancer looks like.

◆   ***Play ball toss*** with your children to help generate a discussion about feelings. The person tossing the ball says a feeling and the person who catches the ball says when they had that feeling. Continue until everyone has had at least three turns.

◆   ***Plant a small garden*** with your children. You can use a variety of things to start seeds in, such as milk cartons, seed starters, or egg cartons. Poke several small holes in the bottom of the container for drainage and add potting soil Have your child plant the seeds in the soil and water with a can that has sprinkle sprouts so the seeds don't wash out. Be sure to get seeds that germinate easily and do not take special care (rye seeds are easiest). Place in a window or another spot that gets a lot of sunlight. Sit back and watch them grow! You can use the garden as a metaphor to talk about what is happening with your illness (see page 12).

◆   ***Have a scavenger hunt*** by asking your children to collect the following things in or around your house within 10–15 minutes:

Shoebox
Dandelion
Lightbulb
Rock
Safety pin
Tree branch (small)
Egg
Quarter
Shoelace
Flashlight

After your children have collected the items above, talk with them about what each item symbolizes related to what you and your family will be going through over the next several months. For example, the egg can represent the beginning of life; the lightbulb can represent hope or insight; the tree branch can represent feelings like going out on a limb, and that everyone needs to be there for each other in case one person falls; the dandelion can represent the weed of cancer; the rock can represent obstacles in the path; the shoelace can represent something that keeps things tied together; a quarter can represent "money in the bank"; and the flashlight can represent something to use to navigate the darkness. You can also choose to add or substitute other items on the list that are important or meaningful to you or other family members.

Write down what the items below symbolize for you and your family. You can add more items to your list discussing what they represent for each of you.

Shoebox

Dandelion

Lightbulb

Rock

Safety pin

Tree branch (small)

Egg

Quarter

Shoelace

Flashlight

CHAPTER TWO

Helping Children
understand treatment

The task of explaining cancer treatment to your children can feel overwhelming. You are likely to be dealing with your own anxiety about treatment. Although many advances have been made in cancer care, the usual first reaction includes feelings of fear and uncertainty about the future. Remember that long-term survival or cure is possible for many people diagnosed with cancer today, so the challenge is how to incorporate cancer and its treatment into a family's everyday life. This includes helping your children deal with the changes it causes.

Understanding Your Responses to Treatment

In order to help your children understand treatment, you will first need to understand your own responses to treatment. The type of treatment you have will depend on the type of cancer, the stage of the cancer, and other individual factors, such as your age, health status, and personal choices. Some people undergoing cancer treatment experience side effects that can be upsetting to children as well as adults. But, there are many things you can do to prevent or control the side effects. Your cancer care team will discuss your cancer treatment with you and will help prepare you for any possible side effects of the treatment.

Remember that many of the side effects are visible ones that your children will be able to see. Some of these include hair loss, nausea, and vomiting. If you experience fatigue, your children will see that you cannot do all the activities that you have done in the past. Children should understand that the side effects are an expected part of treatment, that they are usually temporary, and that they will go away.

Dealing with Your Own Feelings

Facing your own feelings is important in helping your children deal with their feelings. One of the ways children learn to handle their feelings is by watching their parents. You can help your children sort out their feelings by looking at your own.

People cope with cancer in different ways, just like they use a variety of approaches to other life problems. Most people initially feel tremendous emotional upheaval after being diagnosed with cancer. You may experience many painful feelings such as disbelief, shock, fear, and anger. When you are feeling upset, it is hard to absorb all of the information about the cancer. It takes time to accept and understand the diagnosis. After the initial shock of diagnosis and the beginning of treatment, most people come to terms with the reality of living with a diagnosis of cancer. They find they are able to continue their normal lives by returning to work or social activities. Of course there are times when finding strength is hard and the situation feels overwhelming.

Coping and Attitudes

In recent years, a lot of attention has been paid to the importance of having a positive attitude. Some suggest that such an attitude will prevent the progression of disease or the possibility of death. Patients are even told things like, "You'll never beat the cancer if you don't stop feeling sad, pessimistic, depressed," or some other so-called 'negative' reaction. This kind of message is very destructive to patients who, most of the time, are doing everything they can think of to survive.

When people try to deny the very real feelings of fear and sadness, which accompany any serious illness, they miss the opportunity to acknowledge these feelings and learn how to cope with them. Patients who use their energy to stifle legitimate angry feelings often don't have enough of that energy left to cope with life in the here and now.

Hiding feelings will actually keep you from being able to feel hopeful, positive, and more in control of your life. If you keep emotions bottled up, these feelings can lead to more stress and physical symptoms while preventing you from using active coping skills. This may also keep you from getting the help you need.

Many people feel that a real grieving process occurs with a new cancer diagnosis. You will most likely grieve for the loss of certainty in your life. When you face these feelings, it is much easier to work on having a positive mindset about the challenges ahead. Having a positive attitude will make it easier to cope, but developing such an attitude is almost impossible without acknowledging your legitimate grief and anger that this has happened to you and your family.

There is currently no research that proves a positive outlook will guarantee survival or help you live longer. A positive attitude can certainly help you feel hopeful, but it does not mean that you should never feel sad, stressed, or unsure. Trying to keep a hopeful, positive attitude often lessens the impact of cancer on you and your family and may make it easier to solve problems. But it will not make a difference between illness and recovery. Similarly, any difficulty you have coping with your situation will not trigger a recurrence. Those who believe that a positive attitude is the key to their survival may blame themselves if their cancer returns. Cancer is a very complex disease, and people's attitudes don't cause or cure cancer.

Sadness and Depression

Just after learning you have cancer, you may go through a time of grief or mourning. It is normal to go through a period of initial sadness after being diagnosed. You may mourn for the loss of yourself as a healthy person and for the loss of certainty in your life. You may feel hopeless or sad if you see cancer as a roadblock to a life full of health and happiness. It can be difficult to feel optimistic, especially if the outlook for your future is uncertain. Even just contemplating treatment and the time it will take out of your life can be daunting. Your personal history and other things that are going on in your life can also compound feelings of sadness or lead to depression. For example, one patient's mother died on the day she began chemotherapy. She grieved the loss of her mother, but became depressed over her situation, which also included the stress of financial burdens and a recent divorce.

If your emotional upset or sadness is long-lasting or gets in the way of day-to-day things, you may have clinical depression. About one in four people with cancer have depression related to the illness, which causes greater worry and less ability to function and follow medical regimens (see Chapter 3).

What Children Need to Know

After you have had a chance to come to terms with your own reactions to treatment, you will be able to help your children understand their reactions. Children will react in a variety of ways to the changes that you will experience because of treatment. It is important to let them know what to expect during treatment.

Children will usually make a situation much worse in their minds if they are not included in what is happening during treatment. Concealing the truth can require a lot of energy. This energy is better used making sure that children feel safe and prepared for the changes that will take place in the family. Including children in what is happening also makes them feel needed and important. By allowing your children to be part of your treatment and part of your healing, they have a way to be involved and feel needed. This involvement helps build self-esteem.

The goal for parents is to explain treatment in words that children can understand, and to make the needed changes in the family's life to get through a difficult time. Helping children to understand your experience with cancer requires a good sense of timing. Your children may go through the stages you are going through—disbelief, anger, hope, and acceptance. They may have special needs because of their ages. During your illness, their needs may also change.

In general, children need information that will prepare them for what is about to happen to their parent and how it will affect their lives. Use words they can understand. Put yourself in their shoes and tell them about your treatment based on how they perceive the world. For example, tell a teenager about body changes such as hair loss and how you feel about this change. Teenagers are very focused on how they look and sharing your response will make this more real for them. Share enough information so they understand what is happening, but not so much that it becomes overwhelming. Just as when talking about diagnosis, a child's age is an important factor in deciding what and how much you should tell your children about treatment.

How Much Information Is Necessary?

Just as with explaining diagnosis, the amount of information you give your children about treatment depends on a variety of issues, such as their age, personality, and what you have been told about your treatment. You will want to find the right balance between too much information, which could be overwhelming, and too little information, which might raise more questions than answers. After discussing what cancer is and where it is located, children should be told how it will affect you. This discussion should include how their lives may change as a result of your treatment.

In general, young children need less information than older ones and they are more likely to be confused by the information they are given. One mother who talked about surgery for "cancerous tissue" in her lung reported that her children thought she had Kleenex in her body. Children commonly misunderstand the fatigue that is associated with cancer treatment and expect that Mom or Dad will bounce right back after the last treatment, when in reality, this fatigue can continue for many months. It is a good idea to explain that cancer treatment is expected to go on for a period of time, including periods of active treatment in which drugs and or radiation will be given. There may not be new information to report as often as they might expect, but reassure them that you will tell them what they need to know.

If your child does not seem satisfied with the amount of information he or she has, there may be other issues that you may want to discuss with a counselor. Watch your child's behavior. If your child is showing extreme behaviors such as excessive worrying, fighting, not thinking clearly or daydreaming, professional help may be needed (see Chapter 3). Parents usually know how their children normally express being upset. If typical behaviors worsen or if you see major changes in behavior that continues for a long time, there may be problems in coping. Sometimes children cannot find the words to express how they are feeling. Talking with a counselor may give them a chance to express underlying fears or anxiety.

Helping Children Understand Terminology

Children need to understand some basic terms about the disease and treatment.

Biological therapy: treatment to improve the ability of the body's immune system to fight the cancer. Common side effects include fatigue, flu-like symptoms, loss of appetite, and fever.

Biopsy: a piece of tissue is removed from a person's body and looked at through a microscope test to see if a person has cancer and if so, what kind it is.

Cancer: a group of over one hundred diseases in which cells that are not normal grow and divide rapidly. These abnormal cells usually develop into a tumor. Cancer can also spread to other parts of the body.

Chemotherapy: drugs that are used in the treatment of cancer to destroy cancer cells. Common side effects of chemotherapy include temporary hair loss, nausea and vomiting, mouth sores, feeling tired, and increased risk of infections. The kind of side effects a person has depends on the drugs they are taking. All chemotherapy drugs do not cause the same side effects.

Clinical trials: research studies developed to test new cancer treatments.

Malignant: another word for cancerous.

Metastasis: the spread of cancer from one part of the body to another.

Oncologist: a doctor who specializes in treating cancer. Doctors can be medical or surgical oncologists or radiation oncologists.

Prognosis: a predication of what is expected to happen to a person.

Protocol: a detailed plan that doctors follow when treating cancer patients.

Radiation therapy: treatment of cancer with high-energy rays (similar to x-rays) to destroy cancer cells. The side effects of radiation therapy are related to the part of the body being treated. Some examples are reddening of the skin where the radiation is given, hair loss if the head is being treated, nausea if the stomach is being treated, and difficulty swallowing and eating if the head and neck area is being radiated. Fatigue is the most commonly reported side effect of radiation.

Recurrence: the return of cancer cells and signs of cancer after a remission.

Relapse: the same as recurrence.

Remission: the disappearance of cancer symptoms and cells as a result of treatment.

Side effects: problems caused when cancer treatments affect certain parts of the body. Two people with the same cancer or the same treatments will not necessarily have the same side effects.

Surgery: an operation performed to remove cancerous tissue from a person's body.

Tumor: an abnormal mass of tissue.

Talking with Your Children

It is important for your children to know what will happen to you because of your treatment. For instance, people often think that chemotherapy always causes hair loss, but this is not true. If hair loss is a certainty, tell your children so they will not be frightened when it starts to happen. If a parent will be hospitalized, children need to know where, for how long, what is going to happen in the hospital, whether they can visit or at least be in telephone contact, and who will be taking care of them in the parent's absence. If the parent is having surgery, children need to know that the parent will be given special medicines so that it won't be painful. People often feel scared when undergoing treatment, so children should be told that Mom or Dad might be "grouchy" or irritable, during treatment, but it is not the child's fault.

Children will also learn about cancer from a variety of other sources, such as school, television, their classmates, and listening to the conversations of other people. Some of this information is accurate but a lot of it is not. So, children must be able to sort out with their parents what applies to their own situation. Ask your children to tell you what they hear about cancer so you can correct any misinformation. Tell them that everyone responds differently to cancer treatment, so it is not very useful to compare one person's experience to another's.

Children Need to Be Given Information They Can Understand

- Tell them what has happened.
- Explain what will happen next.
- Leave them with feelings of hope that even though you are upset now, there will be better times.
- Assure them they will continue to be loved and cared for.

☙❧

Talking with Toddlers

Since toddlers have developed mentally to the point that "out of sight is not out of mind," they miss and feel a sense of loss when a parent is gone. Having a security object (e.g., a blanket or doll) helps them deal with the situation. These objects represent the safety and security that a parent provides. Most toddlers naturally become attached to some object and keep it with them even when it is ragged or worn. (This was true for Linus and his blanket as shown in the Snoopy cartoon by Charles Schultz.) If your toddler does not have a security object, you might give the child a cuddly toy and suggest that it be used as a reminder of you.

The toddler should be encouraged to grow more independent. Even though the parent is ill and may have a variety of caregivers, the toddler should have as consistent care and rules as possible. Allowing the toddler to explore and play freely will foster healthy development. While things are upsetting in the family, the toddler should not be overprotected. Using dolls or stuffed animals to show different aspects of the cancer illness is one way of helping the toddler know what is going on with the parent. For example, if a parent gets a special intravenous line for medicines, an animal or doll can be used for demonstration. You could tape a straw or tube to the doll and show how medicine goes into the tube to help Mommy get better.

Talking with Preschoolers

Young children think very concretely, so concrete terms must be used in discussing an illness. Cancer treatment can be explained to young children (ages two to six) as a battle between "good guy cells" and "bad guy cells." Taking medicine will help the good guys become stronger so they can beat the bad guys.

Preschoolers will notice and be more affected by the side effects of cancer. Preparing your children can help, but when something finally happens, it can be a shock. Hair loss is a good example. No matter how well you think your child understands that this may happen, if it finally does, expect them to react. Hair loss is such a dramatic event that most people have a negative response at first. Looking in the mirror is a constant reminder that life is not the same. Your reaction as a parent can help. While you may feel devastated about losing your hair it will help if you can balance the situation with a reminder that the purpose of the chemotherapy is to get rid of the cancer cells. Although you look different, it will be worth it if the treatment is successful. Acknowledge that losing your hair is upsetting, but if your children see your acceptance of the hair loss, they will cope better too. Explain to them that the hair loss is temporary. You might say, "Mommy is sick and the medicine she is taking to help her get better is making her hair fall out. That means that the medicine is working."

Vomiting can also be a frightening symptom for children to see. They can provide limited sympathy, but are usually overtaken by their own emotions in response to this problem. Keeping this symptom as private as possible is important. Fatigue is an even more difficult symptom for the energetic preschooler to deal with. They don't understand this symptom and may associate it with pain, which makes them fearful. Careful, simple explanations will be required.

Since children at this age are egocentric (can only think from their own point of view), reassuring them that they have no impact on the cause or course of the illness is important. Remember that children are familiar with being sick, but be careful about saying things such as, "It's like when you had a sore throat and had to go to the doctor." Young children might conclude that the next time their throat hurts, it means they also have cancer.

With the preschooler's need for mastery over play and other skills, the child will feel a part of the family if given a task and told that it will help. For example, your child can draw a picture that you can take to appointments or even for the hospital stay. This can help your child feel important and helpful to you.

Although they are more cooperative than toddlers, preschoolers cannot and should not be expected to be perfect or totally cooperative. As their lives are changed by a parent's illness, they may be less cooperative and act a bit younger. For example, a preschooler who had been getting into his car seat without any trouble may now refuse to do so on a regular basis.

Allowing the preschooler to play as needed, with structure, consistency, and occasional special times, will help the child cope with a parent's illness in healthy ways. A good way of staying connected to your preschooler during treatment is to make audiotapes or videotapes that your child can watch or listen to as needed. This may help ease the loneliness, especially if the affected parent is the primary caregiver.

Talking with School-Age Children

Children who are older (ages six to twelve) are generally interested in more details. By about the age of six, children become very interested in how bodies work. You can explain there are different kinds of cells in the body and these cells have different jobs to perform. Like people, these cells must work together to get their jobs done. Cancer cells can be described as "troublemakers" that disrupt the work of the good cells. Treatment helps to get rid of the "troublemakers" so the other cells can work together once again. Explain the effects of the illness and the side effects of the treatment—such as fatigue, hair loss, weight loss, surgical alterations, and moods—so that the children are not left to fantasize about why these things are happening.

School-age children are quite capable of understanding that their parent may not return to them. This can cause great anxiety and distress. It is important to reassure them that they are not all-powerful or able to control the outcome of treatment. They need to know their behavior cannot cause more illness. Younger children (ages six to eight) have more difficulty distracting themselves from their emotions. They may often feel and express their anger, anxiety, and sadness, so they sometimes need more attention. Because older children have more control over their emotions, you may not be as likely to notice them. But, older children need comfort too, so you'll need to attend to their emotional needs even if they're not obvious.

The outside world is even more important to school-age children. Children who are different (such as those who have a parent with no hair) are often teased and set apart. They may benefit from being around other children who are in a similar situation. They may also benefit by being involved with people outside the family. Distracting activities are even more important for older school-age children. Becoming involved in activities outside the home may help them set other goals, rather than just focusing on the things associated with their parent's illness. They may feel more comfortable talking about their feelings with their coaches, teachers, or other instructors. Sometimes having a professional caregiver talk to children can be very useful.

School-age children are particularly bothered when their parent cannot connect and have fun with them. They may act upset and angry about these changes, and blame the hospital or the doctor. Let your children know that both parents are going to be distracted at times throughout the treatment process. It doesn't mean that you don't care about them or don't love them anymore. Maintaining an interest in your children's activities by encouraging them to bring a momento from a game, videotape of a performance, or project from school will help you to continue to play a supportive parental role. You also may be able to play a quiet game that will involve some interaction, but will not make you feel more fatigued.

Encouraging children to do reports in school on cancer might be one way of both reinforcing the facts surrounding the illness and helping them feel more in control of the situation. Children at this age can also help with simple tasks of nursing care and care in the home. This can help them feel important and valuable.

A child at this age may also act very happy and carefree. Don't be concerned if this is the way your child is acting. This is often how a school-age child will react even if there is a profound change in his life. It doesn't mean that he doesn't have feelings or isn't sad at times.

Talking with Teenagers

Teenagers can fully understand what cancer is and its potential impact on their parents' life. Many teenagers prefer to be treated like adults. They want the facts without any sugarcoating. Some may even want statistics, medical facts, and other health-related information. While older adolescents may thrive on medical details and even do more research on their own to help them cope, younger adolescents (ages twelve to fourteen) tend to not want such detailed information. Too much information can be anxiety-provoking for them.

Children are very conscious of the reactions of others, particularly their peers, who may be very curious about what is happening. For teenagers, this may be even tougher than for younger children. Teenagers are very sensitive about appearances and the possibility of looking foolish. The better prepared they are, the easier it will be for them to accept these changes. Ask them if they know what to say if their friends start asking questions about your diagnosis or treatment. Let them know that you are available to help them feel as comfortable as possible until treatment is finished and life returns to more normal. Since teenagers can be acutely aware of being different, minimizing the differences due to illness will make it easier.

It is tempting to share everything with teenagers because they can understand what is happening. However, their responsibilities should not become overwhelming. Even though teenagers are physically capable of doing a lot, it is preferable not to have them bear too much of the burden of taking care of the ill parent. Such role reversals can be very confusing. While they may be expected to take over some extra activities (maybe cooking a meal or laundry), they should not be overburdened by too many responsibilities. They should be allowed to continue some of their outside activities as well.

Special Issues of Teenagers

Teenagers present special challenges to their families during these years. The developmental task for teenagers is to separate from their parents and begin to define who they are as individuals. Watching teens develop is often a process tinged with worry as they experiment with adult ideas and behaviors, often moving back and forth between the security of childhood and the world of adults. When a parent becomes ill, they struggle with whether to stay and help, or run the other way. In the midst of their ambivalence, family routines change and teenagers might feel that life no longer revolves around them and their activities.

A diagnosis of cancer and treatment means that you are less available to your children, at least temporarily. Other people may be helping out and you may not feel as emotionally connected to your children as you were before. Your energy is divided among many demands such as your family and getting better again. Teenagers can be helpful during these periods because they are capable of assuming some of the household responsibilities. But, the challenge is to decide what they can reasonably do and how to balance this with your teenager's school responsibilities and social life. Monitor how much you are depending on your teenager and recognize the need for open dialogue if this should begin to feel burdensome or overwhelming to your child. Because teenagers are usually not very communicative with their parents and they try to protect them from worry, they might not tell you if things are becoming too stressful.

Teenagers may feel resentful, angry, and confused about what is happening, in addition to their fear that the treatment may not work. Teenagers often experience mood swings, so it is not unusual for them to react to a parent's illness with a wide range of emotions. Sometimes they act out their feelings in inappropriate ways. This can lead to changes in grades and activities at school, problems with sleep, anger, and combative behavior. Teenagers also may appear unfeeling toward either the ill parent or the well parent. Again, this appears to be an attempt to deal with the underlying emotions of the experience. While peer groups are important, teens cannot count on their peers to provide them with the emotional support they need. It can be difficult for them to even share this type of experience with their peers because of the self-consciousness and desire not to be different from others.

Privacy is important to teenagers, so it is important to respect their space. You can't force them to talk about their feelings; however, family meetings are a good way to touch base. Explain to them that this is a chance to review how everyone is doing. Teenagers are particularly sensitive to dishonesty, so it's important to be straightforward. Consider what new information your children might need about your treatment. Evaluate household duties. Do some chores need to be reassigned in light of school demands, or is there a special event coming up that the family should plan for? Who needs special praise for making an extra effort? Family meetings can help family life proceed as smoothly as possible in light of the new demands of cancer treatment.

Teens still need to invest time and energy in their schoolwork and in maintaining their relationships with friends. While maintaining contact with friends may not seem like a priority in light of what the parent is experiencing, these relationships are very important and can offer a teenager much needed relief during periods of stress. Ask your teens how their friends are reacting to your diagnosis. Sometimes teenagers are unsure about what to say or do when a friend has a sick parent, unless they have had experience with illness in their own families. Your teenager may report the same sort of withdrawal that you might have experienced with your own friends who are uncomfortable about your illness. Or the teenager's friends may be asking questions that are uncomfortable to answer or to which there are no easy answers. If this is the case, you will want to suggest ways that your child may deal with these situations, so the teenager is able to maintain normal relationships without too much emphasis on your illness.

Because teenagers are so sensitive about their own bodies, they may also worry that they too might become ill. Or they may worry about inheriting the cancer. Teenage daughters of women with breast cancer may be especially vulnerable to worries about heredity. It is a good idea to discuss these issues with your oncologist so you can give your teenager accurate information.

If your teenagers seem unusually worried or unable to share their concerns with you, check with your hospital about a group for teens whose parents are in treatment or a counselor with special expertise in helping adolescents cope with illness in their families (see Chapter 3).

Ten Ways to Start a Conversation with Your Child

1. How was today on a scale of 1 to 10 (where 1 is terrible and 10 is terrific)? What made it that way?
2. What was the high point (low point) of your day?
3. Tell me the good news and the bad news about school today (work today, practice this week, camp this summer).
4. What's a thought or feeling you had today?
5. What happened today that you didn't expect?
6. (If your child seems preoccupied) I'm wondering what you're thinking about. Would you be willing to talk to me about it?

The following conversation starters
may be especially helpful if you haven't seen
your child for a period of time:

7. Tell me about something good that's happened since the last time we talked.
8. What's something you've done recently that you're proud of?
9. What's on your mind these days?
10. What are you looking forward to these days?

Taking Children to the Hospital or Clinic

Children thrive on routine, so when a parent is hospitalized, they can feel disturbed. If you let your children know there may be trips to the hospital, they will be better prepared to handle the situation. You can explain that it is not necessarily a bad thing to go to a hospital, and that hospitals are places that help people get better.

Surgery can be explained as an operation where the doctor removes the tumor while you are not awake, so it won't hurt. Because the idea of a parent being "cut open" can produce powerful fantasies in a young child, it is important that children be permitted to visit in the hospital as soon after surgery as possible.

In general, it's a good idea to take children to the hospital because it reduces the mystery of what is happening. It provides a sense of reality as well as reassurance to know that you are getting help. Research on children whose parents were terminally ill found that most children were not distressed by hospital visits. The children enjoyed the visits and felt less anxious afterwards.

Most treatment will be in the outpatient setting and it can be reassuring to children to see that nothing bad happens to you when receiving treatments. Plan this kind of visit in advance. Talk with a nurse or social worker who might schedule extra time to spend with your child, explaining what they see and answering questions. You may want to schedule your child's visit on a day when you are able to predict the outcome of the visit. For example, if you routinely feel extremely ill from a chemotherapy treatment, take the child on a day when you are less likely to experience unpleasant side effects.

Visits to an inpatient unit may be more challenging since people are typically sicker when they are hospitalized. It is best to plan such a visit when you feel up to it and can interact with your children in a fairly normal way.

Children should be prepared for what they may see, hear, and feel. Will they see you with bandages and intravenous (IV) bottles feeling and looking sick? Let them know if it is okay to hug or touch you. Sometimes it is a good idea to show children a Polaroid picture to help explain what has happened and how you look. Older children need more preparation than younger children. The trappings of hospital care are often fascinating to younger children, not horrifying as some adults expect. School-age children are very curious about the human body and medical devices. As long as you are able to communicate with a child, a hospital visit offers powerful reassurance that your child has not been abandoned. Again, it is helpful to have a health care professional available to explain the equipment or procedures. Nurses can help children feel comfortable and confident in the people who are providing a parent's care.

Children may benefit by a visit to the hospital even if a parent is critically ill and in the intensive care unit (ICU). With guidance to help them know what to expect, children can cope with the most difficult circumstances. Helping children focus on a positive image may make the visit easier. For example, you can tell them to look at your hand that does not have an IV. Prepare them with what to say to you. Help them make or select a card with a get-well message. Suggest that they tell you about the day. These things help normalize the

Helping Children Cope with Your Hospitalization

Explaining to your children about when, where, and why you are going to be hospitalized will help prepare them to accept the fact that you will be away.

- Explain to your children that the surgery or treatment is going to help you get better.
- Inform them about how long you will be hospitalized. You can give young children a calendar to mark off the days.
- Ask your children to help you pack if they are interested. They can give you something special to take along. Young children can cut out X's and O's (for hugs and kisses) and put them in your suitcase. You can do the same and put them under your child's pillow for them to find at night.
- Call them after school or before bedtime to say goodnight.
- Share tape recorded messages.
- Let them know when they will be allowed to visit and what that will be like.
- When they visit, let them know what they can bring for you (e.g., books, flowers, drawings).
- Some children may be interested in all the things in your room, so you can explain things such as how the bed works, what the call button is used for, and what kind of meals you are served.
- Leave notes or small surprises for children to find while you are gone.
- Children can prepare for your homecoming by making "welcome home" signs.

8003

situation and make children feel more at ease. One nine-year-old boy visited his mother in the ICU and told her about a song he was learning on his trumpet. He thanked the nurse for allowing him to visit and talk with his mom. His dad was able to see the child's strength and continued to help the child understand his mother's illness.

Talking with People at School

Each family differs in the amount of information they want to disclose when a parent is ill. Some people want everyone in their lives to know, while others will tell only close family members. Most people try to strike a balance between the two extremes and tell enough of the outside world so that life does not become more burdensome than it needs to be. Try to think of your child's school as a partner in keeping your child's life as normal as possible. If your child is having difficulty with your diagnosis or treatment, it will probably be evident in his or her behavior, both at home and in school.

Talk with your child's teacher or a guidance counselor. They don't need all of the details about your illness and treatment, just enough to understand that there may be a good reason why your child is acting differently. Some children misbehave, some have trouble concentrating, their grades suffer or they may seem sad or withdrawn. Others may be agitated, or begin to have physical complaints (e.g., upset stomach, headaches, etc.). If these reactions occur in the classroom, you will want your child's teachers or guidance counselor to react appropriately. This involves communicating with you so that together you and the school can help your child cope better.

Your child's teacher will also want to intervene if other children start asking questions about your diagnosis or treatment or in some way make it harder for your child. Children generally do not mean to be cruel, but they are not mature enough to know what is appropriate to talk about openly and what may be private. If the teacher has some basic information, he or she will be able to help answer questions if they arise.

You may want to call your child's homeroom teacher or guidance counselor soon after your learn about your diagnosis. If you explain about your treatment, it opens lines of communication and will help you in the future if your child has problems. Give them guidelines of how much information you want school staff to know. Find out if they have questions. Ask if you could send some booklets to share with other teachers and school staff. If your child has a school nurse, ask to talk to him or her. Ask if you or your partner need to set up an appointment. Many schools have dealt with this kind of issue and may be comfortable to proceed. If a meeting is required, schedule it when you are least tired. Take some booklets with you so you can leave them. Have someone go with you and take notes. The school may have ideas about other resources to help support your child.

Dealing with Emotional Reactions to Treatment

How parents feel can have a big impact on how children respond. People can feel sad or angry when someone becomes seriously ill. This is particularly important when the parent is feeling sick and unable to continue their usual responsibilities. The other parent may be exhausted and perhaps not as responsive to their children's needs as usual. Some children react to this by withdrawing, fearing that they will burden their parents with their own worries. Others may actively misbehave as a way of demanding attention for themselves. Whether the misbehavior is caused by cancer or something else, you still need to do something about it. It is easy to understand that a child may be upset about what is going on, but basic rules of behavior should still apply. Children may feel even more out of control if they perceive that neither parent seems to care how they behave.

As you continue through treatment, your family members will have many worries. Some normal fears are about:
  • losing you
  • not knowing what to do for you
  • not being strong enough when you need them
  • the cancer itself

Their fears may come out in the way they act toward you. They may back away or distance themselves because they find it difficult to deal with the situation, or they may make insensitive comments without realizing it. Your children may become upset when you are unable to continue your normal routines because you are too tired from treatment and you don't feel up to cooking dinner, hosting a birthday party, or going to their extracurricular activities. All of these reactions are normal. Children, like all people, fear and resent what they do not understand. You can help your children by talking to them and keeping the lines of communication open. Working through the activities at the end of the chapter can help with this.

Children usually have a difficult time identifying how they feel when a parent is in treatment. Angry feelings are hard for people to acknowledge, but they are normal when life seems turned upside down. In general, the more honest family members can be with one another, the better. Talking about how you are feeling is one of the best ways to diffuse the tension that families can experience. If you find that you are not as available to your children as you might like to be, think about designating another person, your spouse or other relative or friend, to spend time with your children. Try to talk about treatment in as positive a way as possible rather than focusing on uncomfortable side effects. Tell your children that you are still the same person inside and that you love them just as much as you did before your illness.

Consider ways to help your children express their anger in appropriate ways. They can use toys such as punching bags or kick balls, draw pictures, run, or ride a bike. Some kids like to tear up old newspapers and magazines, while others like to use foam toys to throw against the wall. Pillows can also be used to hit against the bed. Bop toys (usually made to look like cartoon characters) are great for younger children. They are blown up, but have a weight inside at the bottom so they bounce back after being hit. Older children can throw darts against a dartboard. Any activity that does not hurt others and uses up energy is good for releasing anger.

Sometimes when a parent returns home from the hospital, children become afraid and withdraw either physically or emotionally. Younger children (infants and toddlers) seem to adapt better than older children. Parents can prepare children by describing details of what to expect when they return from the hospital. Explain to them whether it is okay to talk to or touch Mom or Dad. Over time, children will adapt to the situation and overcome any fears or reluctance they may have.

How Children May Feel About a Sick Parent

- Some children may feel sorry for themselves when a parent is sick; then they may feel guilty because they think they should feel sorry for the parent instead. Some children will be angry with the parent for being sick and wish the parent was not there—and then feel guilty about that.
- Some children will try to make up for these guilty feelings by being very good and set standards for themselves that are too high to reach.
- Some children will cling too much because they are afraid something will happen to you if you are not there.
- Some children will withdraw from you, trying to become more independent in case something else happens to you.
- Some children will resent the fact that they need to help you when the opposite was true before.
- Some children will laugh and behave badly to cover up their real feelings or their lack of understanding (especially their discomfort in strange situations).
- Some children will act sick to get attention or because they want to be with a parent. They might make a big fuss about a minor illness.

These things will pass with time, but you can let your children know you understand and accept them as they are.

உ௸

Reactions to Uncertainty

Dealing with uncertainty is sometimes the biggest challenge of being treated for cancer. Your natural tendency will be to reassure your children that everything will be fine. Unfortunately, you may not know that for sure until some time has passed. Because cancer can recur or travel to another part of the body, it may be necessary to wait for some time after your initial treatment to know with some certainty what you can expect in the future. For young or pre-adolescent children, this can be quite confusing. Children tend to interpret events by what they see. If your treatment is completed and you are starting to look and feel like yourself again, they will probably assume that the illness is over.

You, on the other hand, probably won't be able to fully relax until you know for certain that the cancer is unlikely to recur (see Chapter 5). You can acknowledge with your children that you are very relieved to have treatment behind you and that everyone is hoping that that will be the end of it. You want everyone to feel hopeful and to get on with their lives. You can promise them that if the cancer should come back, you will tell them what needs to be done at that point. This might mean more treatment, but there's no point in worrying about that unless it happens.

For most young children, this kind of reassurance is all they need to begin putting the experience behind them, especially if you are looking and feeling well. However, some children worry more than others and may need more reassurance. If you think your child is focusing too much on his or her fears, you may want to talk with a professional who has worked with children affected by cancer. Adolescents may be particularly problematic, as they may not be able to openly discuss their fears. Just as parents try to protect their children, children may avoid talking about what frightens them because they don't want to upset the parent. It may be easier for your children to discuss their fears with someone outside the family. A mental health professional can help open a dialogue between you and your children (see Chapter 3).

Coping with Changes

An important factor in coping is understanding what to expect from the illness, the treatment, yourself, and your family. How a family handles cancer is greatly determined by how the family has dealt with crises in the past. Those who are used to communicating effectively and sharing feelings are usually able to discuss how cancer is affecting them. Families who solve their problems as individuals instead of as a team might have greater difficulty coping with cancer.

Everyone in the family will have a different style of coping, and understanding how each family member copes can help you plan for the effects on family life. Some family members may avoid a parent who has cancer because they feel like they have nothing to offer, don't know how to act, or cannot help to make the situation better. Some children may deal with the stress by throwing themselves into schoolwork or hobbies. Others may cope by watching a lot of television or by spending a lot of time outside the house. Although these are ways to escape distress, others in the family can misinterpret them as uncaring or inconvenient.

Almost inevitably during treatment, one or more people in the family have to take over the duties of the person who is ill. Over time, the new responsibilities can create stress. The families that seem to adapt best are flexible about roles in terms of who does what. Cancer can be quite stressful at times, but it is possible to learn effective ways to deal with the changes and uncertainty that you and your family might experience. This is a time to explore what you are learning and examine your abilities. You and your family may find that you will be able to draw upon strengths you did not even know that you have.

Disruption of Routines

During treatment, you may be feeling tired and maybe even sick. You'll also be busy balancing treatment with your other commitments. You may have been the one who "held it all together," but now that you're undergoing treatment, others in your family or support system will need to take on some of your responsibilities. One survivor said, "Your friends and family want to make the cancer go away. But they can't. Letting them help you will make them feel better and you won't exhaust yourself." This added responsibility may sometimes create some resentment, and some family members may even irrationally blame you for your cancer. Much of this is probably due to fear. You can let your children know what to expect during treatment. Keeping your family routines as normal as possible will minimize the disruption in your lives.

To expect life to be the same as it was before a cancer diagnosis is probably not realistic. What you will find is that you and your family will establish a new normal. Regardless of how positive you might be feeling about the treatment, and about advances that have been made, people still experience cancer as a major crisis and feel considerable anxiety about what the future holds. Facing our own mortality and weathering a crisis changes us forever, but children are very resilient, and they will not be traumatized forever. Some people say that cancer has resulted in positive changes for their family. Children can grow in their ability to face other tough experiences in life. They may become more responsible and sensitive to the needs of others. One survivor said, "My children have been my greatest motivation for staying healthy. I think they are more compassionate and sensitive individuals from having to deal with my cancer."

There are ways that people can learn to cope with cancer—the challenge is for people to discover what will work best for their family. With children, one of the challenges is to figure out how they can be involved in the experience without feeling that it is taking over their lives. One of the best ways to accomplish this is to talk about how this experience is affecting everyone and to make a plan as a family about how to deal with changes in family routines. Setting up a regular time for family meetings can be a good strategy if you have not already done so. Such meetings are useful if they focus on everything that is going on in the family, not just the cancer issue. Review what is going on in the family's life, review accomplishments and anticipate any changes that have to be made in people's routines to deal with unexpected events. Making lists of tasks or jobs to be done and assigning these to each family member will help everyone's life run more smoothly. Regular meetings can help the family solve problems before they become overwhelming and can help to relieve tension by bringing concerns out in the open.

One of the best ways to deal with changes in routine and fatigue is to use good time management skills. This is the time to review what is important versus what is "nice" to do. Practice benign neglect and leave some things undone. Be sure that the important things are being done. Don't keep doing the same things over and over. Question habits and routines and make a priority list of what is vital. This way you will have time and energy for spending time with your children.

The actual amount of time you spend with your children is not as important as the quality of the time you spend with them. Consider what activities are the most important to share with your children and what is realistic for you to do. Prioritize your level of involvement in things, such as reading with your children, attending extracurricular activities, helping out with homework, and playing games. Sometimes doing something alone with each child can make him or her feel special.

Setting Limits and Maintaining Discipline

One way of taking care of yourself and taking care of your children is learning how to set consistent limits. It is so tempting to "let go" in this situation and relax the disciplinary standard. But, this is the wrong message for your children. Taking time to set rules and organization for them in a clear, loving, and firm manner helps them feel they are being cared for and safe.

What Children Can Do

- Children often must take on additional chores and responsibilities when a parent is ill or recovering. Provide tasks for them that can help them feel involved and needed during the recovery process when children often feel left out.
- Give small children tasks like bringing in the mail, or painting pictures to send to the hospital.
- Because older children, especially teenagers, may need to help out more than usual around the house, they will need time off and frequent expressions of appreciation.
- Help children keep a routine by having them track their regular schedule and activities and by letting others know what routines to follow. Work with them in jotting down their habits and schedules for meals and favorite foods, regular play dates, sports practices, afternoons at the park, going to bed, and other regular activities.

Kid's Activity Schedule

Activity	Sunday	Monday	Tuesday	Wednesday	Thursday	Friday	Saturday
Meals							
Friends over							
Games and Play							
Practices							
Homework							
Bedtime							

Discipline while you are ill may be difficult because children act up to get the attention they feel they are missing. But a breakdown in discipline can convince a child that something is very wrong at home. It is important to set firm limits and find ways to enforce them—for your sake and for theirs. Communicate your understanding, love, and acceptance of the children but not their misbehavior. Reward good behavior and let them know you especially appreciate cooperation now. Remember it wasn't always perfect before.

Discipline is probably one of the most important things you can maintain while you are ill. It communicates to your child that although there are changes, Mom and Dad are still in control. Discipline should be similar to how it was prior to the cancer diagnosis. There should not be more rigidity and authority than usual.

Having said this, discipline is hard to maintain if the ill person is the usual disciplinarian and if the caregiver tries to pick up this role. Sometimes combining the two parents' discipline styles during this time works. You may have to learn to be understanding and hard at same time—relating to feelings, while maintaining the rules. There can be a fine line between democracy, participatory family decision-making, and family chaos. Maintaining expectations helps children learn a sense of responsibility.

Setting limits with acting-out teenagers is especially important. Because their behavior can have more serious consequences, failing to set limits could have disastrous results. It can be challenging to set limits in a way that is agreeable to them. It is even more difficult in a time-pressured situation that sometimes arises within the cancer experience.

Children are masters at working on their parents' guilty consciences. When you let them down in some way, they are usually not shy about showing their disappointment. But it might be useful to explain to children in the beginning of the illness that you will disappoint them at some point, most likely, with an inability to participate in something in their lives. That way when it happens they will be more prepared for it.

Sometimes the person we most need to reassure is ourselves. You do all that you can do, then let yourself off the hook for the rest. Keeping the long-term healthy picture in mind helps firm the resolve.

Tips for Maintaining Discipline

- Set clear and reasonable limits.
- Be consistent.
- Be flexible.
- Take time to play.
- Provide unconditional love.
- Be aware of your own needs and limitations.
- State clear consequences to misbehavior.
- Follow through with consequences.

 စာ

Friends and Relatives Can Help

Some families are fortunate in having a large network of people to call upon to help. If such a network is not in place, an oncology social worker or nurse may be able to connect families to community resources that can help fill the gaps (see Chapter 3). If there are people who are offering to help, a larger issue may be that it feels uncomfortable to accept. Families that have always prided themselves on taking care of themselves may find coping difficult unless they reach out. Many people are afraid of burdening others and think they should be able to solve all of their problems alone. While you might want to be as independent as possible, dealing with a chronic illness sometimes makes that very difficult. There will be times when the help of others can make a real difference in a family's quality of life.

Examine a week of your children's activities (e.g., getting to piano lessons, being picked up at school, having a sleepover) and decide how a friend, community member, or relative could help. When asking for assistance, be specific about what you want and when you want it. Explain to your friends that you expect them to tell you if the assignment is inconvenient and that they have the right to say no, then you can feel more relaxed about letting them help. Your friends and relatives will feel good knowing they are helping and you can feel less guilty about not being able to continue your activities. Prepare your children for these changes, assuring them that the changes are temporary until you feel better again.

Sometimes friends or relatives unknowingly make things harder because they don't know how to help. Parents may discover their friends withdrawing from them because they are afraid of saying the wrong thing. In these situations, you can reassure your friends that it's okay to ask about your cancer. If you don't want to talk about it, you will tell them. You might also prepare your children for questions and rehearse with them what they might say when people ask about their mom or dad. Questions about a parent's cancer can be upsetting if children are not prepared for the questions.

Recognize Achievements and Special Occasions

Celebrating holidays, family occasions, and milestones such as religious rituals, birthdays, graduations, athletic or academic accomplishments, and steps in the parent's recovery take on increased significance when there's cancer in the family. Continuing to mark important events helps channel energies away from fear and sadness and offers a welcome distraction from the serious concerns that have probably been dominating family life.

While going through treatment may not seem like a time to celebrate, honoring important moments is a way to remember how much you mean to one another, to bolster hope and restore energy, and to confirm that each person in the family is special. You'll see that even if one of you is ill, you have a future as a family. And you can create memories that last forever.

Stay Connected

It's common during treatment for children to feel like their parents don't care about them. Sometimes they feel hurt, rejected, or neglected because they are not getting the attention they are used to getting. Understandably, it is a time when parents can be preoccupied with other concerns. So, it's important to take a few minutes to let your children know that they are still important. Practicing exercises to reduce stress (see Chapter 4) along with your children may be a good way to achieve this.

Hands-On Tools

Helping children deal with the stress of your treatment involves using some of the same skills and activities that helped your child deal with the diagnosis. The activities discussed in Chapter 1 will also work for the stress of treatment. If you did not have your child start a journal, this may be a good time to encourage this activity. Using activities to help your children express feelings is very important. They provide a safe way to talk about what is happening and how cancer is affecting everyone in the family. Not all of the exercises will be right for your children. Use the ones that are most applicable, and adapt them to what works best for your family. Just as with the exercises in Chapter 1, you can use many of the exercises at any time from diagnosis, through treatment and recovery.

◆ *Think of things to do together* that do not require much energy, such as reading or watching television.

◆ *Have clay and other creative materials* to use to work out some frustrations that you and the children share.

◆ *Plan for laughter,* which is good medicine for everything.

◆ *Have your children draw pictures* about the experience of having an ill parent. This is also a good way to express emotions. Or, write a story together about "When Daddy Got Sick."

◆ *Get together with other parents and families* who are coping with cancer. Have your children meet other cancer "survivors."

◆ *Share meaningful poems and songs* that your family has heard before, or they can create their own.

◆ ***Suggest that your children create a strong box*** (like a safe that holds money). You can use a pencil box, purchased box, gift box, or shoebox. Let them decorate the outside of the box through collage or painting. Tell them to place pictures of things that remind them of their strengths on the box. You or a family member may need to help the children identify strengths and tell them this helps with coping. They can use white school glue for the collage. They can use tacky glue if they add objects (like a seashell because they are good swimmers). After the outside of the box is done, tell the children that the inside of the box is for their worries or fears. They may want to draw or write words that express their fears. They may want to cut words from a magazine and paste them on the inside to tell their fears.

Now get them to talk about the inside and outside of their boxes. For the outside, you might help them relate what strength can help them deal with specific stresses. For example, being good in school might help them get information about a parent's illness. For the inside of the box, teach them about feelings. Tell them all feelings are normal and some feelings are hard to have. Placing them in the box helps the feelings to not be so powerful. Note that their strengths will help them cope (just like the box contains their worries). Let them know they can continue to add fears by writing on a piece of paper and placing it in the box. Encourage them to come to you when they want to talk about feelings or have a strong feeling that bothers them.

CHAPTER THREE

Understanding and Using
psychosocial support services

When facing cancer, you will need to sort through a great deal of information in order to understand what is happening to you physically and emotionally. Cancer affects more than your body. It affects how you feel and how you relate to others. Learning how people respond emotionally to cancer puts you in the best position to help yourself and your family.

Cancer is often called a "family disease" because it affects more than the person who is diagnosed. For families with young or adolescent children, this is especially true. Parents have a powerful influence on how their children react to a crisis in the family. Knowing this may seem like a heavy load, but family members can learn how to manage the problems brought about by a chronic illness.

Your understanding of the cancer itself will influence your ability to cope with the cancer. In addition to learning about your illness and treatment, you will want to understand yourself in relation to the experience. Asking for help in understanding cancer and what to anticipate physically and emotionally is not a sign of weakness, but an indication that you want to be an active participant in your life and what is happening to you.

Psychosocial Support Services Can Help People Cope

There may be times during a family's experience with cancer diagnosis and treatment when psychosocial support services can be helpful. These are supportive care services offered by professionals specifically trained in knowing how cancer affects patients and families emotionally. They can offer strategies for solving problems that have a social or psychological basis. By helping people target and prioritize specific issues, they become more manageable and less stressful.

Sometimes people forget they already have skills that have helped them cope with other problems. Psychosocial support services can help people identify the skills that have worked in the past and combine these with new skills to deal with cancer in the family. There are a range of support services available for people with cancer and their family members, such as:

- Financial assistance or counseling
- Individual counseling or psychotherapy
- Play therapy
- Art therapy (see Chapter 4)
- Family therapy
- Group support, education, and therapy for parents and children
- School-based psychosocial services

Cancer is a very complicated disease that requires the help of a variety of specialists. Just as you or other family members have probably required the services of a surgeon, medical oncologist, or radiation oncologist, there may be times when the services of a psychosocial professional may be helpful. These professionals include family counselors, psychologists, social workers, nurses, and chaplains. The use of these services can make a tremendous difference in the family's adjustment to a cancer illness.

How to Know if You Need Help

Your feelings about what is happening to you may be a good yardstick to use in evaluating how you are doing. In the beginning of a cancer experience, most patients go through a period of turmoil, characterized by feelings of anxiety, sadness, and fear about the future. You may have questions about why this has happened to you, the meaning of life in relation to your illness, your relationship to God, along with worries about your job, finances, insurance, and other practical matters. Gradually, as you move through the first stages of treatment, you will be dealing with these feelings and concerns, and hopefully figuring out how to begin addressing them. If you have close relationships with other family members or friends, they will play a part in helping you figure out how to manage the experience. If these concerns are not addressed or you find yourself feeling very sad or preoccupied much of the time or unable to make decisions, it may help to talk with a counselor. The advantage in talking with a professional is that you can find quicker solutions to the problems you are worried about than you would by continuing to struggle on your own.

Your goal will be to gradually feel more in control of the situation and able to devote yourself to managing your treatment along with the concerns of others in your family.

Other family members will have their own concerns as a result of your illness. If you are married, your spouse will be trying to figure out the meaning of your illness in relation to his or her own life. Sometimes couples have a very difficult time talking about a new diagnosis. This is usually because of unspoken fears about the future and how life may be different as a result of the cancer. It is normal to want to protect the people we love from difficulty, but sometimes this results in people feeling very isolated from one another. It is also to be expected that people will sometimes feel angry about what has happened and troubled about having such feelings. Over time, people learn ways of communicating and find safe ways of expressing their concerns. If this process seems to be stuck so that you and your spouse can't figure out how to meet your needs for support, it can be helpful to talk with someone outside of your relationship to gain some perspective.

These issues can feel more burdensome if you are a single parent or you are in a relationship that was already troubled before the cancer (see Chapter 7). Single people may need to identify other ways of getting support. Friends or extended family members may be more important during this time. Or a single parent may want to seek out a cancer counselor or join a support group in order to meet others who are dealing with the same issues.

With troubled marriages or relationships, it may be important to find help so your problems don't interfere with your ability to handle the illness. Dealing with a new cancer diagnosis along with a troubled relationship can feel quite stressful (see Chapter 7). It will be worth it in the end if you can address the issues that are causing your distress. Sometimes people worry that marital disagreements or unresolved stress will interfere with their ability to get well. There is no evidence that stress causes cancer or interferes with positive treatment results. However, it will affect your quality of life and make it harder to cope with day-to-day challenges.

The Influence of Stress on Our Lives

A person's ability to cope and manage stress depends on many things. One way to understand how you cope is by looking at the various physical, emotional, and social influences on your life.

Physical influences include:
- heredity
- hormones
- medical illness

Emotional influences include:
- worries and fears
- depression
- insight and understanding

Social influences include:
- past experience
- family life
- culture
- belief in God or higher power
- finances
- education

Because of all these influences, people vary in their ability to understand themselves and their reactions to stressful experiences. How well you are able to cope is determined by all of these factors.

Symptoms of Distress

Chronic feelings of hopelessness, anxiety, and fear will deprive you of the energy you need to cope with your current situation. So, it is important to pay attention to these emotional signs.

Anxiety

Fear and anxiety are common feelings that patients and families occasionally have when they are coping with cancer. Anxiety may be due to changes in the ability to function in family roles and responsibilities, loss of control over events in life, changes in body image, uncertainty about the future, and concerns about the unknown.

One of the difficult things about anxiety is people may not always know when they are experiencing it. They may think they are just worried. Before they realize what is happening, they are experiencing serious symptoms of anxiety. Sometimes a person may become overly anxious and may no longer cope well with day-to-day life. If this happens, it may be a good idea to seek help outside the family to learn effective coping strategies. Ask your doctor or nurse about your symptoms of anxiety. An assessment can be made to determine the cause of your anxiety and what can be done to treat it.

Depression

Untreated depression accounts for increased health problems in people with chronic diseases like cancer and it is often overlooked. Clinical depression, a treatable illness, occurs in about 25 percent of people with cancer. It causes greater distress, more impaired functioning, and less ability to follow treatment schedules. When your depression is long lasting or interferes with your ability to carry on day-to-day activities, there is reason for concern. Depression can be treated and you should not suffer needlessly when help is readily available.

Treatments for depression in people with cancer include medication (e.g., antidepressants), psychotherapy, or a combination of both, and sometimes other specialized treatments. Antidepressants are prescribed by psychiatrists, primary care doctors, or oncologists who are experienced in their side effects and interactions with other medications you may be taking. These interventions not only improve psychological well being, but also reduce suffering and enhance quality of life.

About Anxiety

What to Look for:
- panicky feelings
- feeling of losing control
- difficulty solving problems
- feeling excitable
- anger or irritation
- increased muscle tension
- trembling and shaking
- headaches, upset stomach, diarrhea, constipation
- sweaty palms, racing pulse

What to Do:
- talk with your doctor about your anxiety and the possible ways to treat it
- talk about feelings and fears that you or family members may be having; it's okay to feel sad and frustrated
- identify the thoughts that may be causing the anxiety
- solve day-to-day problems that are causing you stress
- engage in some pleasant, distracting activities
- seek help through counseling and support groups
- use prayer or other types of spiritual support
- try deep breathing and relaxation exercises several times a day (see Chapter 4)

Do Not:
- keep feelings inside
- blame yourself for feelings of anxiety and fear

Call the Doctor:
- if you are having trouble breathing, are sweating, and feel very restless
- if you experience trembling, twitching, and feeling "shaky"
- if your heart rate and pulse have rapidly increased
- if you have severe problems with sleeping several days in a row

About Depression

What to Look for:

People who have a major depressive disorder have symptoms such as the ones listed below every day for most of the day for at least two weeks.

- persistent sad or "empty" mood almost every day for most of the day
- loss of interest or pleasure in all, or almost all, activities most of the day
- eating problems (loss of appetite or overeating), or significant weight loss or gain
- sleep disturbances (insomnia, early waking, or oversleeping)
- noticeable restlessness or being "slowed down" almost every day
- decreased energy, or fatigue almost every day
- feelings of guilt, worthlessness, helplessness
- difficulty concentrating, remembering, making decisions
- thoughts of death or suicide, or attempts at suicide

If you have any of these symptoms, you should talk with your doctor about your depression and the possible ways to treat it.

What to Do:

- schedule activities that are pleasant
- increase the amount of contact you have with other people
- identify the thoughts that may be causing the depression
- use a problem-solving approach to tackle some of the day-to-day problems that are contributing to your feelings of depression
- seek help through counseling and support groups
- use prayer or other types of spiritual support

How Treatment Can Help:

- it reduces pain and suffering
- it removes the symptoms of depression
- it helps most people feel better and return to daily activities within several weeks
- the earlier you get treatment, the sooner you will begin to feel better

Call the Doctor:

- if you have thoughts of suicide
- if you feel sad, blue, down in the dumps and uninterested in things you used to enjoy
- if you are having trouble breathing, are sweating, or feel restless
- if nothing you do seems to help, even those strategies that have worked in the past

How to Know if Your Child Needs Help

Deciding if your child needs help may feel very confusing as you try to sort out what is a "normal" response to a new cancer diagnosis and what is not. But, parents usually know about their children's behavior and how they typically react to new or stressful situations. While you are learning for the first time how your children react to cancer, you already have experience with how your children deal with other stressful events. Most parents can tell you exactly how each of their children behave when they are upset.

Any family situation that is distressing or that threatens their sense of security is likely to be reflected in children's behavior at home, school, and with friends. Because children, especially young ones, are often unable to talk about how they feel, they show us by how they behave. For example:

- Quiet children may get more silent.
- Rambunctious children may become more agitated.
- Other children may have more trouble separating from a parent.
- Sleep problems may appear for the first time.
- Older children may begin having trouble in school.
- Teenagers may become more distant than usual.
- Some children may begin complaining of physical problems, stomachaches, or may seem fatigued or sad a lot of the time.

It is useful to watch your young children at play. Listen to what they may be saying to their dolls, watch what they are drawing, how they interact with their friends, how easily they can separate from you and so forth. Young children may regress, meaning they seem to go backwards instead of continuing to learn new tasks. Toilet training may be interrupted, children may become insecure and cling to you more, or they may reject your efforts to teach them new ways of behaving. With older children or teens, the same principles apply but these children are better able to talk about their feelings. A simple question like "you seem worried, what's going on?" may help open a discussion. It is natural to assume that all of your children's troubles are related to your illness. Remember that other things in your children's lives are still going on too. A problem with a new teacher, getting invited to a birthday party, and daily activities will still be important to your children.

Children's personalities also affect how they deal with stress. Some children are very "happy go lucky," seem to roll with the punches, and easily adjust to changes in family routines. There are other children whose personalities seem to make things harder. Parents discover early that their children are very different from each other. For example, some babies are very easy to comfort while others cry easily and resist cuddling. These personality traits don't change much as a child grows up; parents learn different ways of behaving to accommodate to each child's personality. So, a child with a "pessimistic" personality may require more patience and help from their parents to see the positive side of a situation.

Look for Signs Based on Age

There are always signs that alert you to the possibility that your child needs help. Look for how extreme the behavioral change is and how long it has been going on. Any deviation from how your child usually behaves may be a clue that your attention is needed. The most important aspect of any warning sign of problems in a child is the degree and duration of the symptom. If the symptom lasts only a day or two, there is no cause for concern. If the symptom continues for weeks or months, some type of outside help may be necessary. The duration of the parent's illness is also a major factor. The longer the illness lasts, the more chronic the stress becomes, which can lead to more significant problems.

Also look for any patterns of small behaviors that may add up to a larger problem. Several subtle behavior changes can be just as important to attend to as one large one. Subtle changes are often harder to detect than extreme ones, so parents should pay more attention to them. Extreme ones will get attention by their very nature. However, behavior is not always an indicator of problems in older children who may be keeping their fears inside. Older children and teens are more at risk for serious depression and suicide.

Infants, Toddlers, and Preschoolers

Play and developmental delays. As a rule of thumb, infants and toddlers should be evaluated every six months for signs of developmental delays (e.g., a toddler who was toilet training that begins to need diapers). This is an excellent time to discuss the family's situation with your child's pediatrician or nurse and review how your child seems to be adjusting.

With toddlers, play situations may provide the most information about how the child is really doing. For example, if a child "loses" or puts away a favorite doll, the child may be concerned about being separated from you. If play is particularly aggressive, the child is likely expressing anger. In conversations with their animals or dolls, is your child focused on the illness or the cancer? When in doubt about a toddler's behavior, it may be best to have a child therapist, play therapist, or art therapist help evaluate your child.

Changes in sleeping patterns. Sleep disturbances are a warning sign in your child. If a toddler doesn't want to go to bed alone when he has been doing so earlier, he may need some extra attention. Setting up a cot in your room or leaving doors open at night with a nightlight might help. Making sure your child gets enough physical activity and keeping to the regular bedtime schedule when possible may dramatically improve sleeping problems. Sometimes giving that extra ten minutes of snuggling time can also improve the feelings of insecurity. If this problem escalates to nightly nightmares, wandering around the house repeatedly in the night, or frequently awakening in distress, professional help should be considered.

Changes in eating habits. Most toddlers have picky eating habits under normal circumstances. Again, noticing the severity and duration are important. If your child refuses to eat for a period of days, there is a problem. Overeating for long periods of time is also a problem. It is important to resist nagging your child about eating changes. Children will eventually eat when they are hungry. Giving children time to adjust on their own may be all that is necessary. Remember that the eating problem is a warning sign and not the primary problem. Getting to the underlying problem is more important. Exercise may also help a child's appetite improve.

School-Age Children

School problems. For the school-age child, difficulties in school help diagnose psychological problems. School-age children may resist going to school, have problems with schoolwork, or develop difficulties in relationships with siblings and peers. For example, a six-year-old boy may have adjusted well to first grade, but after hearing about his mother's breast cancer, may become very clingy and not want to go to school. Visiting the school clinic on a daily basis is another sign of a potential problem. Some children may unconsciously want to be ill so they can be with the ill parent more. Or the child may just be expressing his general distress.

School phobia is more severe. With school phobia, the child has an extreme dread and need to avoid attending school. Unlike adults, a child will not always recognize this fear is unfounded. Younger children will show fear by crying, having tantrums, freezing, and clinging. Children may complain of stomachaches or headaches so that the parent is required to come to school and get them. These behaviors are signs that professional help is needed.

Poor grades or major changes in school performance may be of some concern. These are symptoms of distress in school-age children or teenagers, so you may consider talking with the school counselor. Suddenly giving up treasured after-school activities like sports or the school play may also be a symptom of distress. Sometimes just giving your children permission to do well and continue as they have in the past can help significantly. However, if the problem does not resolve, consultation may be the next step.

Quiet behavior. Children also may become timid in other social situations when this is not their normal behavior. Quiet children are always a concern. They are ordinarily independent, thoughtful, and mature. They tend to keep their feelings inside and perform as usual. These type of children can be more difficult to diagnose because it is harder to tell how they are feeling. Often parents are so grateful that they are behaving at such a stressful time, they accept the behavior without question. If the child, who is normally boisterous, becomes withdrawn and quiet, it is important to ask about the child's feelings. This is true for the normally quiet child as well. You may not have success in trying to tap into those feelings by asking your child directly about feelings. You may need to sit down with your child and play, take the child out to lunch, or go on an outing and wait for the words to come out. Prompting your child to think about his or her feelings is a good idea. The child may not respond the first or second time, but eventually will come forth with feelings. Questions like, "Are you worried about Mom?" or "How has school been going? What was the worst thing that happened today? What was the best?" are good questions.

Fear and anxiety. Fears that children may express at this time can vary greatly. They may be afraid to visit you in the hospital. They may fear being left home alone. They may even be afraid to be near you. Monsters and bad people may become more prominent in their thoughts, conversations, and dreams. Children who fear being lost and never reunited with you may have separation anxiety disorder, which is a condition that involves excessive anxiety about being separated from family or the home. Children with this disorder may often be reluctant to go away to camp or spend the night at their friends' houses. These fears often arise at bedtime. Children may insist you remain with them until they fall asleep. Any kind of separation from parents commonly produces stomachaches, headaches, nausea, and vomiting for children with this disorder. Their dreams are often nightmarish tragedies that involved fire or other catastrophes. Fears about death and dying can be part of this syndrome, particularly about themselves. These symptoms must last up to four weeks to be diagnosed as separation anxiety disorder.

Fears should be taken seriously and not belittled or treated lightly. It is certainly appropriate for older children to fear the parent's death and progression of illness. Fear is most significant if it occurs as a major change and impacts the quality of life of the child or family.

Depression. A feeling of powerlessness or helplessness in a difficult situation can trigger depression in some children. Children who have a history of depression in their families are more at risk for depression. Depression in children under the age of thirteen is not common. While children do feel sad and sometimes worthless, it is more difficult to determine depression in children who are unable to talk about their feelings. Younger children express depression with physical symptoms like headaches or stomachaches, loss of appetite, being more irritable, acting tired, and withdrawing from interaction with other children. Other signs of depression in younger children include irritability, temper outbursts, and restlessness. If a sad mood keeps your child from participating in usual activities, there is cause for concern. If symptoms last for several weeks in a row and interfere with functioning at home or school, you should consult your doctor or nurse.

Suicidal Behavior

If your child is acting depressed, and talking about suicide, he may be sincerely asking for help. If your child says things like, "I just don't want to be here anymore," or "You make me so mad, I'm going to kill myself!" take it seriously. No one can afford to be too cautious to prevent a tragedy. It may be tempting to think your child is just being her dramatic self. Instead, tell your child how sad it makes you to hear that, and seriously explore that with him or her.

What if your child seems to be making such a statement just to see your reaction? Or what if your child makes such statements repeatedly? Here is where your knowledge of your child comes into play. If the child has that gleam in her eye that looks like, "I've got him where I want him," it's possible she is manipulating you. A child who is seriously depressed does not rebound quickly from feelings of sadness. The feelings last and are not easily dismissed.

School-agers or teenagers who act recklessly, but may not actually talk about suicide are also at risk and need professional help. For example, a child who knows better may dart out into traffic, or a teenager may drive very fast and dangerously. Any behavior that involves breaking the law or destroying property is a cry for help. Taking drugs and drinking alcohol are other warning signs that warrant extra intervention.

കൈ

Teenagers

Anxiety and helplessness. Because teens are more aware than younger children of cancer news in the media and are able to think about the future, they may be extremely frightened of death and loss. They may feel very alone and abandoned. Older adolescents are more capable of empathy, so they may feel overwhelmed by your pain and their own helplessness in dealing with it. As a result, some may become aloof, while others may become anxiously over-involved in your care.

Poor judgment, problems in school, physical complaints. Some more mature teens cope as adults do, by seeking and evaluating information and turning to friends and counselors for help. However, some may act out aggressively and destructively or begin to fail in school, even if they've been trying to keep up. Some may start developing headaches, rashes, and other physical problems.

Depression. Mood swings are common among teenagers. They often go through periods of irritability, oversensitivity, listlessness, and apathy. It can be difficult to tell when a teenager is depressed, and depression in teenagers often goes unrecognized and untreated. If you notice any of the following symptoms lasting for several weeks, there may be cause for concern:

- sad or agitated moods without any periods of happiness
- loss of interest in activities
- fatigue
- drop in school performance
- withdrawal from friends
- personality change
- problems with eating or sleeping
- frequent comments of despair
- excessive acting-out behaviors
- persistent feelings of worthlessness
- thoughts about suicide or preoccupation with death

Other distress signals. Excessive drug or alcohol use, sexual promiscuity, eating disorders, violence with peers and authority figures, and self-mutilation are all ways that some teenagers demonstrate their difficulties with life experiences. Teenagers often have little realization of the powerful emotions behind such self-destructive behaviors and actions. Overachievement, withdrawal, and perfectionism are other ways they may try to manage out-of-control feelings.

> Any significant changes in behavior that last for more than a couple of weeks are **WARNING SIGNS** that a child is having difficulty. If a child starts talking about wanting to die or suddenly begins giving away favorite possessions, seek help from a mental health professional immediately.

When Things Are Not Getting Better

Additional attention from parents may be all that young children may need to adjust to the situation. Family support is crucial in helping them deal with problems. Talk to them, try to get them to verbalize their feelings, and always express your love. Kids need to know that the parent who is not ill will be there to take care of them.

When problems continue or are destructive to the child or to others, you or other responsible adults must intervene. Always try to determine your child's understanding of the illness. Despite your best attempts, your child may have imagined something that is deeply disturbing. This may be true even for older children.

Even with less severe problems, talking to the school guidance counselor or seeking help through the social work or psychosocial department at your hospital or through other resources is a good strategy. It can relieve the pressure on you when your own capacity to cope with your children's reactions is limited.

If the usual methods of handling problems are not working and your child is becoming more and more unhappy, upset, or distressed, professional help may be the answer. Children who were having problems before will probably have a worse time now, so counseling may be needed to help them manage their increased distress without long-term consequences for their schoolwork and peer relationships.

It can be useful to talk with your child's pediatrician, school counselor, or with the counseling staff at the hospital where you are receiving treatment. Since these people have experience with how other children have reacted to illness in the family, they may be able to offer a useful way of looking at the problem. They should also be able to refer you to mental health professionals who have experience with children whose parents have a chronic illness. Support groups, individual, and family counseling can also be helpful (see pages 79–89). You can also ask about support groups just for children of parents with cancer. See the Resource Guide in the back of this book or ask your doctor for recommendations.

Asking for Help Can Be Difficult

For many people dealing with a cancer diagnosis, sorting through medical decisions is an enormous challenge. You may not have the energy to cope with much more, so you may ignore emotional issues or put them off until later, when life feels more settled. This is understandable because people can only cope with so much at one time. However, where children are concerned, problems don't usually disappear.

One of the important concerns for people needing support services is how they feel about asking for help. Some people have the idea that they should know how to handle every emotional problem that comes up even though they have never been confronted with a crisis like cancer. Sometimes people feel that needing help with a problem is a sign of weakness. This is not true. In fact, asking for help can be a sign of strength. Getting support from others can help you solve problems quicker than attempting to solve them alone. Helping your children develop ways to cope with your illness will teach them that while we cannot control everything that happens in life, we can control how we choose to deal with problems.

It is good to ask for help early in order to prepare for the challenges of treatment. During periods of active treatment, you may feel too tired and overwhelmed to seek help. In addition to your physical needs, family members will have their own reactions and worries. If family problems are worrying you, it may be harder for you to feel in charge of the situation. By enlisting help early in the process, you can be sure your resources are close at hand.

In addition to their worries about a sick parent, your children are coping with other concerns and stresses. They are expected to continue to meet expectations in school, manage relationships with siblings and friends, and keep up with chores at home and other responsibilities. They are also growing and changing in the ways they think about life and themselves. It can feel like a difficult task to help your children manage the challenges of your illness. Asking for help and learning how other families have dealt with these problems can help preserve your energy and guide your children through a difficult time.

Health care professionals want to help families maintain a reasonable "quality of life" in the face of cancer treatment. This means making good choices about managing the illness, preserving your hope for the future, and taking charge of the situation. What you don't want to have happen is to feel victimized by the disease or feel that the disease has taken over your life. You will always have choices about how to feel and what to think about the situation. With your help, your children can also learn how to deal with cancer and its treatment.

For some people, the idea of getting professional help for emotional or family problems is not acceptable. They feel that somehow needing help means that they are "weak" or that it's a sign they are unstable or even "crazy." It may seem to you that some people sail through the cancer experience, never revealing any stress or difficulty dealing with a problem. People make judgments about themselves and say things like "what's wrong with me that I cannot seem to cope with my problems?" Or, "I should be able to just 'tough it out' until the trouble passes." While we all have this tendency to feel we should be able to manage just about anything, there will be times in this experience that toughing it out just does not work.

When dealing with a diagnosis of cancer, it may not be possible to control everything going on in your life. This is new territory and it will take some time to discover what works best for your particular family. Don't be hesitant or afraid to seek the support you need in order for you and your family to begin to feel better.

Many Services Are Available

Making a decision about what is best depends on a number of factors, such as what services are available from your hospital or community, cost of services, and how your reaction to the cancer is affecting your children. For example, if you are feeling sad or depressed, it may be hard to find the energy to respond to your children. You may be feeling too worried to deal with all that is going on. Talking with a counselor may help you put a new perspective on the situation and find ways to solve problems that you may not have considered. Often feeling more in control of your own feelings and reactions may be all it takes to help your children get back on track. Counselors are also more objective and can help children express feelings in a way that parents cannot. If you feel that you are coping with your illness and treatment reasonably well, but your children seem distressed, consider meeting with a counselor who is experienced in how children react to a parent's illness.

Individual Counseling

Individual counseling offers an opportunity for you or your child to talk with a counselor. The counselor will ask questions about you and your family and about what is worrying you. Finding out how you have dealt with problems in the past, including what is or is not working now, will be useful in knowing how to help you. The counselor will help you prioritize your needs so your biggest concerns can be addressed first. You may talk about different ways to approach the situation before deciding what to try first. It is important not to get impatient or frustrated if your first approach doesn't seem to be working. Problem solving is often a stop and go process. You may try out a variety of possibilities before arriving at an approach that is right for your family. With individual counseling, a therapist can help you develop a plan with goals to:

- resolve the immediate crisis
- improve a problematic behavior
- improve coping skills
- improve social skills
- resolve conflicts
- prevent hospitalization or things getting worse
- maximize family and other support

Counseling is also available specifically for children. As the child's parent, you will be involved in your child's counseling either by meeting with the counselor along with your child, or by having periodic meetings to familiarize yourself with your child's progress. Counselors who specialize in helping young children often use play therapy to understand what is worrying them. For teenagers, talking about problems is usually what is offered. Don't expect that your child will be happy with the idea of counseling. People usually have trouble accepting the idea that they might need to change the way they think or behave. Teens especially may resist getting help because of the nature of adolescence. Feelings of uncertainty about who they are as people along with their suspicion of adults may make it hard to convince them to try counseling. But just as we do not let children play in the street, we cannot allow the child to decide against counseling. One of the most valuable aspects of individual counseling is that the person who receives the therapy has someone who can confirm their pain and suffering.

Play Therapy

Traditional therapy that involves talking is sometimes not effective with children because they often lack the words to express their feelings. Play therapy is another avenue for helping children express their thoughts and feelings. Play therapists listen and respond to children's play to help them express and work through their concerns. As children play, they bring out problems and learn ways to master them. So children feel more in control and stronger emotionally.

When children are stressed by a family member's cancer, they can work out how to deal with their stress through play. For example, a therapist may take a child into a playroom with carefully selected toys. The child picks out the toys and the therapist observes and interacts with the child at play. For example, a child may "play" doctor with an animal, and even act out the animal getting a bone marrow transplant. In the process of doing this, the child could discuss feelings about the animal being sick and fears that the animal might not get well. In the hands of a professional therapist, the play is interpreted for parents so that strategies for helping the child can be planned. The child, through play, may symbolically "heal" the parent and gain comfort from these activities.

Play therapy can also be focused in a particular area, such as helping a child to be more cooperative in the family. In this situation, children in a group can pretend they are a family and the therapist may encourage the child to learn more helping skills.

Another form of play therapy that includes the whole family is called filial play. Here, the parents are taught to conduct a play session with their children. This type of play can strengthen family relationships and is more efficient because it can be easily done within the home.

Art Therapy

Art therapy can be an excellent way of helping children express their feelings (see Chapter 4). Art therapists have studied the significance of specific colors or how things are arranged in a child's picture. Their interpretation of children's art can be invaluable in providing clues to what is going on inside the child. In a safe and non-threatening environment, an art therapist invites children to use simple art materials to communicate their concerns. In the process, children express feelings they often cannot put into words. They may increase their self-esteem and confidence in the process of this expression. Hopefully, the art therapy can make the feelings more accessible so they eventually can communicate verbally.

How to Plan Counseling for Your Child

The following are suggestions to use when planning counseling for your child:

- Talk with your child about your own feelings of distress when you see him or her hurting.
- Talk with your child about the behavior that you see that concerns you.
- Give your child some choice about who to see. A school counselor may be easier to accept than a complete stranger.
- Ask your child to try one or two sessions before making a decision.
- Enlist the help of a relative that is close to your child.
- Use the analogy of a cancer doctor helping with cancer, a throat doctor helping with a sore throat, a counselor helps deal with feelings.
- Reward your child for going through a first session by discussing how proud you are. Spend some extra time with your child in casual play or going out to dinner.
- Don't ask for details of the sessions, but get a general sense of how it is going.
- Stress that counseling is always confidential and that the counselor would need your child's permission to discuss what is going on with a parent. (If a person is suicidal, the usual norm of confidentiality does not apply.)

If you are still unsuccessful in getting counseling for your child, try getting help for yourself. You may find your child or teenager is more willing after you have made some changes in how you are interacting with them.

Family Counseling

Some professionals think family counseling is the best way to cope with cancer because a diagnosis of cancer always affects other family members. Families who have been affected by cancer struggle with difficult issues at different times. They may be more troublesome now for longer periods of time and your attempts to change things or to feel better may not be working. In the typical family with its mixture of different personalities and ways of behaving, change is often difficult. Recognizing a problem and understanding why you or family members behave in a particular way are important steps in figuring out how to get along better.

Family counseling can decrease the feelings of isolation family members sometimes experience. It provides a forum for interaction and allows people to feel less helpless because they are actively doing something to deal with the illness. Talking about the problems can actually make them more manageable. Some sessions can also be held without the parent who has cancer, which sometimes allows other family members to talk about scary or painful feelings more openly.

A family counselor will understand how the behavior of individuals affects the family as a whole. The problem may be the way family members communicate with one another. Or it may be a lack of understanding among family members about behaviors that are hurtful or get in the way of people receiving support from each other. Sometimes tension in a family will prevent people from understanding each other so the same hurtful behaviors continue. It is often easier for someone outside the family to help family members look at a situation differently and try new ways of behaving so that they can help and support each other.

Is Family Counseling Right for You?

One of the ways to decide about family counseling is to look at what is going on in your family. Ask yourself some of the following questions:

- Can I talk to my spouse about how I feel?
- Is my spouse or partner able to listen to what I am saying or does it seem to be too painful for them?
- Does it help to talk to my spouse when things are going badly?
- Do we always end up in a fight about how we expect each other to be reacting?
- Do my children seem worried a lot?
- Do they tell me how they feel?
- Are my children misbehaving more than usual?
- Is it harder to get them to listen?
- Do my children seem sad or lonely?
- Do they seem unable to enjoy being together as a family?
- Are they fighting among themselves more often?
- Are their grades suffering?
- Am I getting more complaints from my child's school?
- Are my children backsliding in their development? (For example, are they having more difficulty separating from you, maintaining toilet training, being unable to play by themselves or being unusually dependent on you?)
- Is my family able to accept help from others?
- Do I resent that people outside the immediate family seem happy?
- Do I feel angry a lot of the time that others don't have this burden to deal with?
- Are financial or insurance problems interfering with my ability to deal with my family?

Support Groups for Parents

The purpose of a support group is to help people share their concerns with others and to learn new ways of solving problems. Support groups often instill hope and enable people to overcome feelings of helplessness. Research has shown that people with cancer are better able to deal with their disease (e.g., greater toleration of cancer treatment and treatment compliance) when supported by others in similar situations. Support groups can also help relieve stress, confusion, and fatigue.

Participants can also expect to learn more about the disease itself in addition to getting new ideas from others like themselves. For instance, a newly diagnosed person who has never had to share a diagnosis with children can hear from others how children might react. A woman with breast cancer can learn from other women about breast reconstruction. Young adults can hear how others have approached problems with dating from those who have "been there."

Support groups for people with cancer can be organized in several different ways. Some meet in hospital settings, within a community agency, a family service agency, or even in a patient's home.

Talking Increases Intimacy

One couple went to a family therapist at the wife's request following her mastectomy and chemotherapy. She was worried that her husband thought she was ugly and that he was afraid to touch her. In the counseling session, he was able to express his real fear about her dying and of hurting her physically. As they listened to each other, they realized the problem was that both had feelings and thoughts they were not expressing. Not talking about the effect of the surgery led them to become distant and tense. As they were able to be more open, their marital distress improved.

ೲ

Open-ended groups are set up to allow anyone with cancer or their family members to attend, often for an indefinite period of time. Or, people might attend during periods when the course of the illness is changing, decisions need to be made about new treatment options, or new family concerns arise.

Closed groups are those in which the same group of people meet for a prescribed period of time. They can be organized for people with the same diagnosis, the same sex, the same stage of disease, or by the kind of treatment people are receiving.

Groups can be organized by topics where different issues are discussed each week or month. Others may have a free-flowing agenda where participants can discuss whatever topic they choose. Regardless of the kind of group you attend, confidentiality should be discussed by the group facilitator at your first meeting. You should feel free to discuss your concerns with others and know that what is discussed will remain confidential.

Either professionals or cancer survivors may lead groups. Professionals include oncology social workers or nurses, psychologists, psychiatrists, psychiatric nurses, marriage and family therapists, or clergy (see pages 91–92). Professionals should be licensed in their respective fields and have skills in group "facilitation." This means they will have had training in how to go about setting up a group and how to help members get their needs met. They also know how to deal with group members who tend to monopolize the conversation or with people who are so upset or angry that a group is counterproductive. If a cancer survivor is facilitating a group, that person may or may not be able to accomplish these tasks. Some cancer survivors are very comfortable dealing with difficult behaviors and have had enough life experience to be very effective in a group setting. Others may not, or may find themselves getting uncomfortable or overwhelmed by what is being discussed in the group. Feel free to ask about the credentials or certification and training of group leaders.

People often have strong feelings about the kind of group they want. Some will feel that only someone who has had cancer will make a good group leader. Others want a professional who might be able to offer more education about cancer or emotional issues. You might consider trying both types of groups to identify what type is right for you. Your "comfort level" is usually a good indication. If you feel comfortable sharing your feelings and are better able to address your problems, the group will probably be helpful. If not, consider another group or another kind of counseling until you figure out what is best for you or your family.

Some people are more comfortable in groups than others. It may be easy to imagine sharing your feelings with others or it could seem like a real invasion of your privacy. There are very few "rights and wrongs" with regard to how people feel about participating in a group. Some people find them very useful at the point of diagnosis or changes in treatment because there is so much information to sort through in order to make a decision. Patients with more experience with cancer can help new patients know what to expect and how to avoid situations that may be troublesome.

It may take time to determine how much of yourself to share with others. Some group members will be very talkative while others learn better just by listening. Usually, group members will gradually feel more comfortable in discussing their concerns and will get satisfaction from helping others in the group. You should never be forced to share in a group.

The nature and seriousness of your needs will help you decide whether to try a support group. Some needs lend themselves to being addressed in a support group. Examples are the need for information, such as how children typically react to a parent's diagnosis, how to explain your diagnosis at work, or how to communicate better with your doctor. Other problems, such as severe marital or psychological problems, may seem too "private" to share with others.

The intensity of your feelings about a situation will also help you to decide about attending a group. You may feel so upset about your situation that the idea of discussing it with others makes it worse. Your own or your family's distress may make it impossible to listen to anyone else's problem. In fact, there may be times when the danger of feeling more overwhelmed is too great to consider joining a group. For people struggling with these kinds of feelings, or serious marital conflict, an individual counselor can concentrate on you as an individual and help you feel more in control. Once you feel less anxious or overwhelmed about your situation, you will be in a much better position to benefit from a support group.

Support Groups for Children

Sometimes children try to behave like adults so that life will be easier for their parents. A support group for children gives them a safe place to air their frustrations and ask questions (e.g., "Did your mom or dad's hair fall out?"). There is a growing awareness that children of adult patients can benefit from support groups and in fact, have many of the same needs as adults. The primary need is to meet other children whose parents have cancer. Children can feel very isolated if a parent is sick and think no one else has the same feelings and worries. Cancer is different from other problems that children experience. For example, most children know other children whose parents are divorced, but they are less likely to know other children whose parents have cancer. This can make them feel very alone and different from their peers. When children meet other children in this situation, it is comforting to realize that others have the same worries, such as:

- Why does my parent have cancer?
- Is it something I did that made it happen?
- Did my parent "catch" cancer from someone else?
- Will my other parent get sick?
- Can I get cancer?
- How will my life change?
- Will my parent still be able to take care of me?
- Will my friends at school know about Mom or Dad's cancer?
- Should I talk to my friends about it?
- Will people treat me differently?
- Will my parent die from cancer?
- Who would take care of me if that happens?
- Will I still be able to do things I enjoy?
- Will Mom or Dad still do "fun things" with me?
- Will I have to take care of Mom or Dad?

Support groups for children should be lead by professionals. People like schoolteachers or guidance counselors, art therapists, music therapists, oncology social workers, or nurses who have experience with children are examples of possible group leaders. The professional should be knowledgeable about cancer and the issues it raises for families. Parents can check with resources in their community to find support groups for children whose parents have cancer (see

Resource Guide). Hospital social workers, nurses, psychologists, clergy members, and school counselors are good resources to ask about support groups in your area. Some cancer treatment centers offer support groups for children, although they are less available than groups for adults.

The success of a group for children will depend on the professional's use of play therapy or activities to involve children and address tough issues. Adults receive help by talking about a problem, whereas children are less able to verbalize their feelings and worries. The professional should be experienced in getting children to open up through play, drawing, and games. A cancer survivor sometimes is able to do this if he or she has had experience or training in working with children in groups and knows how to safely talk about uncomfortable feelings.

The best kind of support program for children is one that offers a corresponding group for parents. Parents are a child's best teachers and you will learn from other parents about ways to deal with your children. Parents should expect feedback from the group facilitator about their child's participation in the group and what the professional thinks about the family's needs.

At first, your child may not be excited about the idea of attending a support group. People usually resist doing something new, and children are no exception. Once your child experiences the support and fun a group offers, he or she will probably be quite eager to participate.

What to Look for When Choosing a Counselor

How to Choose a Counselor for Yourself

The two most important factors to consider when choosing a counselor are a person's experience in helping people deal with cancer and how comfortable you feel with that person. People who work in cancer treatment centers tend to have more knowledge and experience with emotional responses to cancer than counselors who work outside of a cancer facility. A counselor's experience with cancer is important because it offers a way to understand how your reactions and feelings are related to your situation. For example, an experienced cancer counselor will know that a newly diagnosed patient might become depressed after treatment is completed (see Chapter 5). This is because the medical facility symbolizes safety and the treatment is fighting against the cancer. Once the treatment is over, parents may find they are more worried than they were when they were "doing something" to control the disease. A cancer counselor will recognize that this is a normal response for many parents and can help you deal with this. However, if your depression is long lasting or you find that talking about your feelings is not helping, a cancer counselor might suggest a trial of an antidepressant medication to help you get back on track.

Another important factor to consider in selecting a counselor is the person's professional training or credentials. At a minimum, professionals should have a master's degree in one of the counseling fields along with appropriate certification and/or licensure. While credentials will demonstrate a person's formal education in their chosen field, they ideally should be combined with their experience with cancer. You should not feel shy about checking all of this out. Professionals who are secure in their abilities know that people need to find the most knowledgeable source of help and should not be reluctant to give you this kind of information.

Sometimes people feel that unless a counselor has had cancer or has "been there," he or she will not be able to help. While a personal experience will certainly add a dimension to the counselor's expertise, it's important not to underestimate the value of experience with other parents and families. Even if a counselor has never had cancer, we have all experienced life crises and losses of one kind or another. A personal experience is only one criterion to consider in evaluating the suitability of the counselor.

Always pay attention to how you feel with the person you are seeing. Does it feel safe to share your concerns with this person? Do you trust the counselor's ability to help you? Do you feel that the counselor is really able to listen to you and understand you as an individual? Do you think your family could relate easily to this person? This may be hard to understand or describe. However, trust your instincts. If somehow you just don't feel comfortable after a few sessions, it would probably be wise to try someone else. You will know when you have found the right "match."

You should also know that counseling may not always make you feel better at first. Counseling sessions may feel uncomfortable in the beginning because of all the issues that are brought to the surface. If you have been trying to forge ahead without thinking about the problems, it can be difficult to face them head-on. But in the long run, it pays off to address them because you can learn better ways to cope.

Types of Mental Health Professionals

There are a variety of professionals that offer mental health services. Counselors often come from the fields of social work, psychology, psychiatry, pastoral counseling, or psychiatric nursing.

Social workers help patients and families adjust to the practical and emotional problems related to illness. They focus on social functioning, which includes helping people with community and financial resources, health care systems, employment concerns, legal and ethical issues, insurance coverage, childcare, and other needs. Oncology social workers specialize in helping people manage concerns related to cancer and work closely with health care professionals who treat people with cancer.

Psychologists are licensed professionals who usually have doctoral degrees (Ph.D., Psy.D., Ed.D.) and provide counseling and psychotherapy, testing if needed, consultation, and outreach. They may also do research and teach. Psycho-oncologists are psychologists or psychiatrists who are experienced in counseling people with cancer and their loved ones. They can help people adjust to illness, manage anxiety and depression, and cope with other emotional problems.

Psychiatrists specialize in the field of medicine that focuses on the diagnosis and treatment of mental illness. Psychiatrists are licensed doctors (M.D.s) who can prescribe medication to treat psychiatric illness. They can also conduct psychotherapy.

Marriage and family therapists are mental health professionals trained in couples counseling and family therapy. They are licensed in many states to work with people who have problems in their relationships, marriages, or families. They have graduate training (a Master's or Doctoral degree) in marriage and family therapy and at least two years of clinical experience. If your state does not offer licensure, inquire if the therapist is certified in marriage and family therapy from the American Association for Marriage and Family Therapy (AAMFT).

Licensed professional counselors provide mental health and substance abuse counseling in a variety of settings. They are licensed in many states to work with individuals, families, groups and organizations. They have a master's degree (or above) and are trained in understanding human growth and development, and psychosocial problems.

Pastoral counselors focus on spiritual beliefs for psychological healing and growth. Certified pastoral counselors have mental health backgrounds and religious training.

Psychiatric nurses conduct assessments of patients' psychosocial and physical needs; offer assistance with basic life skills; and provide individual, group, and family counseling, training, and education. They are trained and certified as nurses who specialize in mental health services.

How to Choose a Counselor for Your Child

Child therapists are trained to know about normal childhood development and how to evoke responses from children in a specific way. Many of the same criteria that you would use in choosing a counselor for yourself apply to finding a counselor for your child. Specific training and expertise in working with children is the most important criterion. Ask about training or certification beyond the counselor's basic education. Consult with the counselor by phone or in person. Try to get a "fit" between your child and the counselor. Ask friends and professionals to make referrals. If someone does not feel right to you, listen to your gut.

At the first session, establish clearly the counselor's way of operating. Find out how confidentiality is handled. Be sure you are comfortable with the level of information that will be shared. The first session should involve talking with you as well as your child and doing an in-depth assessment.

How to Know if Counseling Is Working

You will know if counseling is helping you and your family by asking the following questions:

- Are you gaining more insight into the nature of your difficulty?
- Is it becoming easier to "see the forest for the trees"?
- Do you feel like you have more options?
- Do you feel less sad, anxious, or worried?
- Has your concentration improved?
- Is it easier to make decisions?
- Do you have a clear idea where you are going, or what needs working on immediately and what can wait until later?
- Are you more in control over how you are feeling and behaving?
- Has your performance improved (school, home)?
- Can the counselor give you some idea of how long you will need help?
- Can you tell your doctor how counseling is helping?

If the answers to these questions seem positive, you are probably on the right track. If you don't feel good about your answers to these questions, discuss them with your counselor. If the relationship with the counselor doesn't feel comfortable or trusting, it may be that you expect different things from the therapist, or you misunderstand the counseling process in some way. Or you may need to find someone who is a better "match" for your personality or situation. This takes work but your, and your family's, quality of life is well worth the effort.

∞

Finding and Paying for Services

The availability of support services will depend on where you are receiving your treatment. In cancer centers, universities, or community hospitals in urban areas, these services are likely to be available. Smaller community hospitals or those in more rural areas may not offer all types of services. In this situation, you may find the services you need from agencies in the community, (e.g., wellness centers or community mental health centers), private counselors, or peer support programs.

In a large institution or cancer center, a team of people, including doctors, nurses, social workers, rehabilitation specialists, and nutritionists usually deliver cancer treatment. In some treatment centers, a social worker, clinical nurse specialist, clergy person, or counselor may be available to help with family issues. Usually they start with a "psychosocial assessment" to identify the needs of your family. This does not mean they think you won't be able to cope with cancer—it is a way for you to be understood in the most comprehensive way. Health care professionals understand that cancer is a complex disease with the potential to cause great family stress. For this reason you may want to learn what services are available. Where children are concerned, just learning about some of the issues from people who have worked with other families in similar situations may be helpful. In some hospitals, your doctor or nurse may refer you to the department that offers counseling or psychosocial support services. You can also refer yourself or ask where you can find this kind of help. You can also get valuable referrals by "word of mouth" from people in schools, churches, adult learning classes, and others in the community.

Insurance

Insurance may pay for counseling services. This will depend on your particular health plan and its coverage for mental health services. Most health plans have some coverage available for counseling but often, this is more limited than it is for medical services. Legislation is being considered to achieve mental health "parity" meaning that coverage for mental health services should be as available as coverage for physical illness. However, this is not universally accepted by the insurance industry, so you may find that your coverage is inadequate for your needs. Some policies only pay for a limited number of sessions or if it is a managed care policy, it may limit your choices about who you can see. Your insurance may have "contracts" with certain mental health providers, but not with others.

If you are having trouble understanding your coverage, ask the hospital or clinic social worker to help. If counseling services are not available free of charge where you are being treated, they can usually help you to get accurate information about your plan and what is covered. They also know about services in the community that may operate with a sliding scale adjusted to your income. The hospital billing department may also be able to examine your policy and determine your coverage.

Keep track of your bills and submit them as soon as you receive them so you know when you have reached the limit for reimbursement. Hospitals, clinics, and physicians' offices usually have someone who can help you complete claims for insurance coverage or reimbursement.

You may not have any trouble getting claims covered by your insurance company, but if any of your claims that should be covered are denied, ask for help from your doctor's office or from personnel at the hospital claims office. Sometimes the company denies claims based on specific language in the policy. To figure out if the denial is due to an interpretation of the policy, ask the company for the specific language that supports the denial of coverage. To find out what the appeal process is, call your insurance company. If you feel you have been treated unfairly by a private insurance company or a health maintenance organization (HMO), contact your state insurance commission.

You should get the kind of help you need when you need it. Don't feel embarrassed about needing support services. Most people need help at some time in their lives in dealing with a life situation. You will learn a great deal about cancer as a result of having the experience. Give yourself the opportunity to learn what you will need in order to manage the impact of cancer for yourself and for those you love.

CHAPTER FOUR

Taking Care
of yourself

Many parents struggle with balancing their own needs and the needs of their children. Because you may not be feeling well or your time may be consumed with schedules for treatments and doctor's appointments, it can be difficult to provide your children with enough attention. This can lead to frustration and guilt, especially since children may actually become more demanding at this time. However, researchers have found that parents are more effective when they have taken care of their own needs. This chapter offers a variety of ways you can take control of your own sense of well being so you can feel more relaxed and focused.

Therapies to Soothe Your Mind, Body, and Spirit

The following exercises or therapies involve some form of physical or mental relaxation, and you may find they can help you better deal with the emotional stresses resulting from the effects of treatment or pressures of responsibilities at home. You have the power to change how you respond to stress by practicing many of these techniques. In general, all of these therapies promote healing, improve mood, and enhance the quality of your life. Whether you are reading this book as a parent who is ill, or if you are the well parent, these exercises can be valuable. Many children will also find these exercises enjoyable.

Books, videos, and web sites offer information on many of these different techniques. You can usually find a class on some of these methods at fitness and community centers in your area. Some hospitals and health centers offer training in these techniques. If these are not enough to help you cope, consider taking advantage of the various psychosocial support services that are available (see Chapter 3).

Expressive Therapies

These techniques involve harnessing the healing power of the arts (visual, performing, and literary) and creative expression. Expressive therapies are used as a way of identifying and expressing feelings. They tap into experiences on many levels through the senses including verbal, visual, hearing, and touch. They are particularly valuable in helping children access unexpressed concerns. A variety of methods are used, such as drawing, clay, sand play, music, writing, storytelling, drama, dance, and fantasy play. Several expressive therapies are highlighted below.

Art Therapy

Art therapy involves the use of creative activities to express emotions through the many media of the visual arts (see Chapter 3). Using clay, paints, crayons and collages, you can create a painting, drawing, mask, sculpture, or other art pieces that express your feelings about cancer. Using art provides a way for people to come to terms with emotional conflicts, increase self-awareness, and express unspoken and often unconscious concerns about their cancer. This therapy views the creative act as healing, which helps to reduce stress, fear, and anxiety. Art therapy may also be used to distract people whose illnesses or treatments cause pain.

Many medical centers and hospitals include art therapy as part of inpatient care. Art therapists work with people individually or in groups. The job of the art therapist is to help people express themselves through their creations. Although uncomfortable feelings may be stirred up at times, this is considered part of the healing process.

Dance Therapy

Dance therapy is the therapeutic use of movement to improve the mental and physical well being of a person. It focuses on the connection between the mind and body to promote health and healing. Dance therapy is based on the belief that the mind and body work together. Through dance, it is thought people can identify and express their innermost emotions, bringing those feelings to the surface. Some people claim this can create a sense of renewal, unity, and completeness.

Dance therapists help people develop a nonverbal language that offers information about what is going on in their bodies. The therapist observes a person's movements to make an assessment and then designs a program to help the specific condition. The frequency and level of difficulty of the therapy is usually tailored to meet the needs of the participants.

Dance and movement are great stress relievers for children. Children are less inhibited than adults in using their bodies to express feelings. Children may make up a story to go along with their dance to express feelings they are not aware of having.

Dance therapy is used in a variety of settings with people who have social, emotional, cognitive, or physical concerns. It is often used as a part of the recovery process for people with chronic illness. Dance therapists work with individuals and groups, as well as entire families.

Journaling

Consider keeping a journal. Writing down your experiences and your emotions can help you come to terms with your situation. You might use your journal to reflect on the impact of cancer on your life. It's also a way to express any feelings of anger, confusion, joy, or guilt in a healthy way. A journal should not be a burden or something you feel you have to do. It may even help you keep up with symptoms and treatment. When writing in a journal, do not worry about grammar or complete sentences. You may even find that you doodle or draw notes in your journal. Use a computer to journal if it is easier for you. Remind your family that a journal is private. You may find that you want to share certain parts to help express yourself to others. You might even want a trusted friend or counselor to comment on certain passages. Gaining insight into your thoughts and feelings will help you cope.

Feelings Journal

Acknowledging your feelings and working through them is a healing process. Being honest with yourself and others and giving yourself permission to feel and express negative feelings is usually the most helpful thing to do. You can complete the sentences below to help you explore your reactions to many of the situations you are likely to face.

When I first found out I had cancer, I felt

I wish that I

I can make this come true by doing

One of the things that I worry about most is

What would make me feel better is

When I tell others about my condition

I feel closest to people when

Other people see me as

I would like other people to see me as

When I get angry

When things get to be too much, I

I would like to handle things by

I couldn't get along without

The best times are

What I like most about myself is

Music Therapy

Music therapy is a method that consists of the active or passive use of music in order to promote healing and enhance one's quality of life. There is some evidence that when used along with standard treatment, music therapy can help to reduce pain and anxiety and relieve chemotherapy-induced nausea and vomiting. It may also relieve stress and provide an overall sense of well being. Some studies have found that music therapy can lower heart rate, blood pressure, and breathing rate. Some medical experts believe it can aid healing, improve physical movement, and enrich a person's quality of life. There is some evidence that music therapy reduces high blood pressure, rapid heartbeat, depression, and sleeplessness.

Music therapists design music sessions for individuals and groups based on individual needs and tastes. Some aspects of music therapy include music improvisation, receptive music listening, songwriting, lyric discussion, imagery, music performance, and learning through music. Individuals can also perform their own music therapy at home by listening to music or sounds that help relieve their symptoms. Music therapy can be conducted in a variety of places, including hospitals, cancer centers, hospices, at home, or anywhere people can benefit from its calming or stimulating effects. Many rehabilitation departments employ music (art and dance therapists) to help people recover from physical problems caused by cancer therapy.

Other therapies based in the arts have similar benefits. Music and dance therapy provide outlets for feelings and improve mood and well being. Children may especially enjoy creating songs or dances with a parent. Children enjoy picking out songs that are relaxing or restful to them. Popular artists who have wonderful albums for children include Kenny Loggins and Art Garfunkel. Music by native American artists using flutes and similar instruments can be soothing and help children go to sleep at night.

Mind, Body, and Spirit Techniques

Aromatherapy

Aromatherapy is the use of essential oils—fragrant substances distilled from plants—to alter mood or improve health. Aromatherapy is promoted as a natural way to help people cope with chronic pain, depression, and stress, and to produce a feeling of well being. Some evidence suggests that these effects may be real.

There are approximately forty essential oils commonly used in aromatherapy. These highly concentrated aromatic substances are either inhaled or applied as oils during massage. Essential oils should never be taken internally. Also, people should avoid exposure for a long period of time. You can apply the oils yourself, or they can be applied by a practitioner. Many aromatherapists in the United States are trained as massage therapists, psychologists, social workers, or chiropractors who use the oils as part of their practice.

Children enjoy working with herbs and the smells in the oils. You may want to ask your child if he would like to try some of these activities. These are practical ways to use the scents and oils in your daily life. You may want to allow your child to pick out a favorite scent. Let your child rub the oils on your hands and on himself. This activity allows your child to support you and becomes a wonderful bonding time. If your child is having trouble sleeping, both of you may want to make a good dreams sachet to put under the pillow. Fill a small cloth pocket with dried lavender. You can explain that lavender helps give "sweet dreams" to children and adults. Place the lavender under your pillow. You can also note that the sachet is a symbol of your caring for each other.

Biofeedback

Biofeedback is a treatment method that uses monitoring devices to help people consciously regulate physiological processes that are usually controlled automatically, such as heart rate, blood pressure, temperature, perspiration, and muscle tension. It has been approved by an independent panel, convened by the National Institutes of Health (NIH), as a useful complementary therapy for treating chronic pain and insomnia. It can also regulate or alter other physical functions that may be causing discomfort.

With the guidance of a biofeedback therapist, patients use various monitoring devices to measure information that controls their bodily processes. Patients can adjust their thinking and other mental processes in order to control bodily functions, such as heart rate, temperature, perspiration, blood flow, brain activity, or muscle tension. The process is repeated as often as necessary until patients can reliably use conscious thought to change physical functions.

Hypnosis

Hypnosis is an effective tool for reducing blood pressure, pain, anxiety, nausea, vomiting, phobias, and aversions to certain cancer treatments. It is a method of putting people in a state of restful alertness that helps them focus on a certain problem or symptom. People who are hypnotized have selective attention and are able to achieve a state of heightened concentration while blocking out distractions. This allows people to be open to images, suggestions, and ideas for resolving issues and improving their quality of life. Hypnosis is one of several relaxation methods that have been approved by an independent panel, convened by the NIH, as a useful complementary therapy for treating chronic pain.

There are many different types of hypnotic techniques. However, most hypnosis begins with an induction. While a person is sitting or lying quietly, the hypnotherapist talks in gentle, soothing tones, describes images, and

Hypnosis Exercise for Children

Because children move easily between the real world and the pretend world, they can use hypnosis to help them go to sleep or deal with scary times. Parents may use techniques from self-hypnosis to teach their children to relax when afraid or worried. If you are comfortable, tell your child you are going to teach some magic. Explain that this magic will work when your child is afraid or tired. You can start by asking your child to breathe in deeply like sucking on a straw then blow out like blowing up a balloon. As you talk, keep your voice slow and soft. Invite your child to relax with you—don't command. Tell your child to do this and notice how relaxed your child's body becomes. Next, ask your child to listen and count backwards with you. Tell your child when you get to one you will tell a story. Now begin counting with the number ten, and between each count, encourage your child to breathe slowly. You may use the directions given in the relaxation exercise below. When you get to number one, tell your child to look around a see a wonderful magical door. Use your imagination to create a story about a land that lies behind this door. After about ten minutes, tell your child that it is time to come back from the magic land. Count forward to ten and when you reach the number ten, tell your child to awaken and be refreshed (or fall into a natural and restful sleep).

repeats a series of verbal suggestions that allows people to become relaxed, yet deeply absorbed and focused on their awareness. People under hypnosis may appear to be asleep, but they are actually in an altered state of concentration and can focus on a specific goal.

Contrary to what many believe, people under hypnosis are not under the control of the hypnotherapist, nor can they be made to do something they wouldn't ordinarily do. Hypnosis is not brainwashing, and ideas are not "planted" in people's minds to make people do things against their will. Quite the opposite is true. Hypnosis is used to help people gain more control over their actions, emotions, and bodies. People who practice hypnosis are licensed. It is important to be hypnotized by a trained professional. People can also be taught how to hypnotize themselves.

Imagery and Visualization

Visual imagery is a relaxation technique that involves mental exercises designed to enable the mind to influence the health and well being of the body. Some people with cancer have found that imagery can reduce nausea and vomiting associated with chemotherapy, relieve stress, enhance the immune system, facilitate weight gain, combat depression, and lessen pain. Imagery and visualization are also useful to help decrease anxiety about tests and procedures that you may undergo. Using imagery to relax will keep your veins from constricting when you are having an IV injection or infusion. Imagery is also very helpful for children who are having trouble going to sleep.

There are many different imagery techniques. One common technique, guided imagery, involves visualizing a specific image or goal to be achieved and then imagining achieving that goal. Athletes often use visual imagery to help improve their performance.

Imagery techniques can be self-taught with the help of books or learning tapes, or they can be practiced under the guidance of a trained therapist. Imagery sessions with a health professional may last twenty to thirty minutes. The more you practice these exercises, the more you will be able to reduce your stress.

Children can easily be taught to use imagery and visualization techniques since they usually have active imaginations. This can also help them talk about and deal with their fears and insecurities about cancer in the family.

Visual Imagery Exercise

Choose a quiet place with minimal distractions. These exercises may be done sitting up or lying down. Try to get as comfortable as possible, but do not cross your arms and legs because that may cut off circulation and cause numbness or tingling. You can close your eyes at any time. If you choose to keep your eyes open, fix your gaze on one spot in the room and continue to stare at it throughout the exercise. You can ask someone to read the instructions to you or you can record the instructions for yourself.

Allow your attention to shift to your breathing. Breathe in through your nose and out through your mouth. Breathe slowly and deeply from your diaphragm. Continue to take deep, comfortable breaths. Do not force your breath, just observe your slow, steady, rhythmic breathing. With each breath, allow yourself to breathe more slowly and deeply. Each time you exhale, relax your muscles and imagine that you are blowing away all your tension, anxiety, fear, or confusion. Each time you inhale, imagine you are taking in healing breaths of relaxation. You can choose a word, idea, or image to help you deepen that feeling of relaxation as you continue to breath deeply. If any distracting thoughts come to mind, just let them drift away and focus your attention on your breathing.

Now let yourself go to a very relaxing place. Choose a place where you feel most calm and most at peace. Imagine going down six steps and at the bottom of the steps you move into this very relaxing and peaceful place. Notice everything around you in this place. Notice all the sights, smells, and feelings that are there. Let yourself be absorbed and comforted in this special place. This is where you feel safe, whole, and protected. Experience this feeling deep in your muscles, your skin, your bones, and throughout your body. You may sense your body becoming still, like the surface of calm water that reflects the sky. You may experience a sense of warmth like being embraced in a soft blanket. Allow yourself to take in all the comforting feelings as you enjoy your special place.

After you take a few moments to enjoy your relaxing, healing place, gradually let yourself walk back up the six steps. You can always go back to your special image or place, it will always be there for you. But, for now, it's time to come back to this place where you will carry your comforting feelings within you. Begin by counting backwards from six and working your way back to the top. *Six, five*–you're becoming more aware of the sounds around you in the room. *Four, three*–feeling more alert, awake, and refreshed. *Two, one*–you are now back in the room feeling deeply relaxed, but alert and ready to face the rest of the day. Slowly open your eyes if you haven't already.

Massage

Massage involves the manipulation, rubbing, and kneading of the body's muscle and soft tissue. It has been shown to decrease stress, anxiety, depression, insomnia, pain, and relax muscles. Many people find that massage brings a temporary feeling of well being and relaxation.

There are many different massage techniques. Massage strokes can vary from light and shallow to firm and deep. The choice will depend on the needs of the individual and the style of the massage therapist. If a person has a particular complaint, the therapist may focus on the area of pain or discomfort. Typical massage therapy sessions last from thirty minutes to one hour. Massage should be conducted by a trained and licensed professional.

Some massage therapists are trained in parent/child massage. If you have one in your area, this might be a good stress reliever for you and your child. It could be a great way to show your caring of each other.

Meditation

Meditation is a mind-body process that uses concentration or reflection to relax the body and calm the mind in order to create a sense of well being. It is a relaxation method approved by an independent panel, convened by the NIH, as a useful complementary therapy for treating chronic pain and insomnia. It may help people with cancer control pain, decrease stress, and improve quality of life.

Meditation can be self-directed, or guided by doctors, psychiatrists, other mental health professionals, and yoga masters. The ultimate goal of meditation is to separate oneself mentally from the outside world. Some practitioners recommend two fifteen- to twenty-minute sessions a day.

Prayer and Other Spiritual Practices

Spirituality is generally described as an awareness of something greater than the individual self and is usually expressed through religion and/or prayer. Studies have found that spirituality and religion are very important to the quality of life for some people with cancer. Intercessory prayer (praying for others) may be an effective addition to standard medical care. The benefits of prayer may include reduction of stress and anxiety, promotion of a more positive outlook, and the strengthening of the will to live.

Proponents of spirituality claim that prayer can decrease the negative effects of disease, speed recovery, and increase the effectiveness of medical treatments. Religious attendance has been associated with improvement of various health conditions such as heart disease, hypertension, stroke, colitis, uterine and other cancers, as well as overall health status.

Many medical institutions and practitioners include spirituality and prayer as important components of healing. In addition, hospitals have chapels, and they contract with ministers, rabbis, and voluntary organizations to serve the spiritual needs of people with cancer.

Relaxation Exercises

Relaxation exercises are used to manage anxiety, reduce muscle tension and fatigue, relieve pain, increase energy, and enhance other pain relief methods. Relaxation exercises can be learned through tapes and books that are widely available, which provide step-by-step instructions for a variety of relaxation techniques.

There are many different types of relaxation techniques (including visual imagery as mentioned earlier). Progressive muscle relaxation is a relaxation technique that increases the awareness of how to identify tension in the body and the ability to relax specific muscles groups throughout the body. Deep abdominal breathing involves learning how to breathe from the lower part of the abdomen. Many people breathe from the chest rather than the abdomen, which is less effective in creating a state of relaxation. Slow rhythmic breathing begins by staring at an object, or closing the eyes and concentrating on breathing or on a peaceful scene. Autogenic training is a technique used to teach the mind and body to respond to positive messages that are repeated to oneself. Autogenic phrases help people to monitor themselves by focusing their awareness on the connection between verbal commands and physical relaxation. The relaxation response by Herbert Benson, M.D., is a form of meditation that involves sitting comfortably in a quiet place and repeating a mantra silently.

Tai Chi

Tai chi is an ancient Chinese activity that was introduced to reverse the tenseness that came from practicing the martial arts. It was developed to help the warrior relax and not be on the offensive all the time. The purpose was to

Relaxation Exercise

Many people with cancer have found relaxation techniques helpful. These techniques can be used anytime—even for short periods of time. Practice relaxation once a day, but not within an hour after a meal since digestion may interfere with the ability to relax certain muscles.

1. Sit quietly in a comfortable position (such as in an easy chair or sofa) and practice this exercise when you are not feeling rushed.

2. Close your eyes if you feel comfortable doing so.

3. Deeply relax your muscles, beginning with the face and going throughout the entire body (shoulders, chest, arms, hands, stomach, legs) and ending with the feet. Allow the tension to "flow out through your feet."

   Now concentrate your attention on your head, and relax your head even further by thinking, "I'm going to let all the tension flow out of my head. I'm letting go of the tension, and I'm letting warm feelings of relaxation smooth out the muscles in my head and face. I'm becoming more relaxed."

   Repeat these same steps for different parts of your body: your shoulders, arms, hands, chest, abdomen, legs, and feet. Do this slowly—spend enough time to feel more relaxed before going on to the next part of the body.

4. When your body feels very relaxed, concentrate on your breathing. Become aware of how rhythmic and deep your breathing has become. Breathe slowly and deeply. Breathe through your nose. As you breathe out, say the word "calm" silently to yourself. Slowly take a breath in. Now slowly let it out and silently say "calm" to yourself. Repeat this with every breath. It helps you to relax more if you concentrate on just this one word "calm." Continue breathing deeply, becoming more and more relaxed.

5. Continue this exercise for ten to fifteen minutes. Remain relaxed and breathing slowly. At the end of the exercise, open your eyes slowly to become adjusted to the light in the room, and sit quietly for a few minutes.

   When it is over, ask yourself how relaxed you became and if there were any problems. One problem can be drifting and distracting thoughts. If this happens at the next session, think to yourself, "Let relaxation happen at its own pace." If a distracting thought occurs, let it pass. Let it fly away like a bird. Don't fight it. Concentrate more on the word "calm." Let the thought drift by and repeat "calm" over and over again as your breathing gets slower and deeper—as you relax more and more.

6. Do these exercises regularly—once a day is best. In the beginning, it may help to have someone else give you the instructions. You can record these instructions on an inexpensive tape recorder and play them when you are relaxing. If you prefer, you can record yourself giving the instructions and use that.

7. When practicing, choose a time when you will not be disturbed. Tell the other people in your household what you are doing and ask them to be quiet during the exercise.

8. After you become skilled at this exercise, you will find that it is easy to apply when you are getting tense. For example, if you are feeling tense while waiting to see the doctor or for a treatment, you can easily close your eyes for a few minutes and use this exercise to relax and feel calm.

9. It's a good idea to learn this relaxation technique early—before anxiety becomes severe. It can then help to keep severe anxiety from happening.

mediate the effect of the martial arts on the inner self, especially the effects of anger. It is a mind-body, self-healing system that uses movement, meditation, and breathing to improve health and well being. Tai chi is based on the philosophy of Taoism, a Chinese belief system first developed in the sixth century B.C. Its slow, graceful movements, accompanied by rhythmic breathing, relax the body as well as the mind. Tai chi relies entirely on technique rather than strength or power. It requires learning a number of different forms or movement groups.

Research has shown that tai chi is useful as a form of exercise that may improve posture, balance, muscle mass and tone, flexibility, stamina, and strength in older adults. Tai chi is also recognized as a method to reduce stress and lower heart rate and blood pressure.

People who practice the deep breathing and physical movements of tai chi claim that it makes them feel more relaxed, agile, and younger. This general sense of well being is said to reduce stress and lower blood pressure. Practitioners claim it is particularly suited for older adults or for others who are not physically strong or healthy.

Tai chi is taught in many health clubs, schools, and recreational facilities. Practitioners believe that daily practice is necessary in order to get the most benefit from tai chi. Once an individual has mastered a form, it can be practiced at home.

Yoga

Yoga is a form of nonaerobic exercise that involves a program of precise posture and breathing activities. It can be a useful method to enhance a person's quality of life and help relieve some symptoms associated with chronic diseases such as cancer, arthritis, and heart disease, and can lead to increased relaxation and physical fitness.

People who practice yoga claim that it leads to a state of physical health, relaxation, happiness, peace, and tranquility. There is some evidence showing that yoga can lower stress, increase strength, and provide a good form of exercise. Proponents also claim that yoga can be used to eliminate insomnia and increase stamina.

There are different variations and aspects of yoga. The most common form of yoga involves the use of movement, breathing exercises, and meditation to achieve a connection with the mind, body, and spirit. The goal of yoga is perfect concentration to attain the ancient Hindu ideal of *samadhi*—separation of pure consciousness from the outside world through the development of intuitive insight.

Practitioners say yoga should be done either at the beginning or the end of the day. A typical session can last between twenty minutes and one hour. A session may include guided relaxation, meditation, and sometimes visualization. It often ends with the chanting of a mantra (a meaningful word or phrase) to achieve a deeper state of relaxation. Yoga requires several sessions a week in order to become proficient. Yoga can be practiced at home without an instructor, or in adult education classes or classes usually offered at health clubs and community centers. There are also numerous books and videotapes available on yoga.

Cognitive Therapies

Cognitive techniques focus on helping people gain a sense of control over the way they think about things. Such strategies seek to change patterns of negative thinking, replace irrational ideas, ease worries, and reduce mental stress.

COGNITIVE RESTRUCTURING TECHNIQUES				
SITUATION	**FEELINGS**	**THOUGHTS**	**EVIDENCE**	**ALTERNATIVE RESPONSE**
Explain what happened that was upsetting	Describe how you felt after it happened and the intensity of the feeling (1=weak, 10=strong).	Write down any negative things you told yourself or thoughts you had.	Is there any validity to the irrational beliefs? Provide examples.	Write down other things you can tell yourself to counterbalance the negative thoughts.
• *I was late and missed my appointment*	• *Stupid (8)* • *Frustrated (6)*	• *I never do anything right.*	• *That's not true. There are a lot of things I do right.*	• *I am usually on time.* • *Next time I will be on schedule*

Cognitive Restructuring

This is a method that helps people change faulty thought patterns. Cognitive restructuring techniques involve identifying negative thoughts, feelings, or fears and replacing them with constructive or realistic ones. These strategies are based on the theory that what leads to emotional consequences is not what happens to you in life, but how you interpret it. The techniques help you review your habitual ways of responding to stress and modify your coping style by thinking through the problem differently.

There are many different kinds of cognitive restructuring techniques. Identifying critical thoughts and irrational beliefs is the key to understanding how to change these patterns. You can teach yourself to develop an internal dialogue and change any automatic negative thinking into rational responses. One way to do this is to record your negative thoughts, list how they make you feel, and write a rational response to the situation.

Distraction

One of the easiest and most useful coping methods for handling short-term discomfort is the use of distraction. If you have ever daydreamed in a meeting, counted sheep, worn headphones to avoid the boredom of exercise or a bus ride, or kept busy to avoid thinking about something unpleasant, you are an old hand at distraction. Distraction involves a wide range of techniques, from imagery and thought stopping to watching or listening to music, movies, and tapes. The goal is to direct your awareness away from the physical or emotional distress you are feeling. This technique does not require much energy, so it may be very useful when you are tired. It can be used to manage anxiety before surgery or treatments, control nausea or vomiting, handle acute (short-term) pain, manage treatment-related phobias (e.g., fear of needles or MRIs), or stop repetitive, negative thoughts.

Any activity that occupies your attention can be used for distraction. If you enjoy working with your hands, crafts such as needlework, model building, or painting may be useful. Losing yourself in a good book might divert your mind from the pain. Going to a movie or watching television are also good distraction methods. If your concentration is diminished, try math games, like subtracting 47 from 1,000, or counting back from a certain number. Slow, rhythmic breathing can be used for distraction as well as relaxation. You may find it helpful to listen to relatively fast music through a headset or earphones. To help keep your attention on the music, tap out the rhythm or adjust the volume. If the mere smell of the hospital's chemotherapy wing makes you ill, you can distract yourself by taking along a small bottle of perfume or a scented oil to smell when you feel nauseated.

Graded Task Assignments

This method is used to identify a goal and then to list small steps to achieve it. For example, the demands of treatment can make it difficult to keep in touch with friends. When your treatment is over, you'll want to resume these friendships but may feel overwhelmed by the task of trying to rebuild your life.

First, identify your goal: to reconnect with your support system. Then give yourself graded task assignments—specific, manageable steps toward that goal. You might make a list of people with whom you've lost touch and then call one friend a day. The next tasks might be to make one lunch date a week, to go on that date, and to talk with a friend about how things are going. Step by step, you can reach your goal without exhausting yourself physically or emotionally.

Thought Stopping

Cancer raises many fears and it is hard not to worry about everything from your physical health to medical expenses, work, and family pressures. But constant worrying can hinder your quality of life and healing efforts. The technique of thought stopping is a tool used for many years by behavior therapists and psychologists. It is a simple self-help tool that is used for interrupting repetitive or unpleasant thoughts.

First, identify the thought you want to stop (e.g., "I'm not a good parent," or "How will I ever get through this?"). Then, every time you have this thought, visualize a big red stop sign (or another image that means "halt" to you) and say "Stop!" loudly and firmly to yourself. Some people wear a rubber band around their wrists and snap it every time the intrusive thought arises. Practice this exercise until it becomes automatic. Then whenever the thought pops up, so will the image, and your inner voice will silently command the thought to stop.

CHAPTER FIVE

The Time
after treatment

Life Returns to a New Normal

After you have finished your last round of treatment, you begin looking toward the future. You and your family, relieved and overjoyed, celebrate your successful treatment. Things can now return to the way they used to be, right? No, things will never be exactly the same again, but you will establish a new normal.

For most cancer survivors, the end of treatment is a time of transition and adaptation. You may be adapting to physical changes while you are still struggling with lingering effects of treatment, such as fatigue. You and your family may also be facing unexpected emotional upheaval and fears about the future. Your children may have trouble readjusting and expressing their feelings now that you have completed treatment.

The fact that things can never go back to the way they used to be does not have to be a bad thing, however. You can learn how to live being a survivor—even how to thrive at it. Life after cancer will be challenging in many ways for you and your family, but it can also bring new opportunities for closeness, understanding, and a powerful appreciation for life.

What to Expect After Treatment

Coping Once More with Change and Uncertainty

Now that treatment is over, you and your family will be going through yet another transition period, as you adapt to life after cancer. You may come home from your last cancer treatment anticipating the happiest moments of your life, only to find yourself more upset and afraid.

Everybody in the family may be struggling with how each person's role has changed because of cancer. Some family members may feel angry about what the disease has put them through. In fact, it's normal for family members who have supported you during your illness to "let down" and feel safer in expressing some of their own needs and frustrations, now that you're getting well. Or, your family may be unwilling to let go of your role as a sick person. They may continue to protect and indulge you although you're ready to regain your independence and responsibilities.

This time of transition can be an opportunity for you and your family to grow together. Relationships will be put to the test, and it may feel like a bumpy transition for everybody at times. But, you may find that you and your family can grow closer than ever before as you work together toward solutions in the period after your treatment.

Feeling a Void After Treatment

Over the past few months you have established a routine for clinic visits or hospitalizations and developed relationships with your cancer care team. Things that were extremely disruptive in the beginning became regular occurrences in the course of treatment. Visiting your doctor helped you to feel your health was being monitored, and that you were being taken care of. What is familiar can be comforting, and when you begin making fewer visits to your treatment center, you may feel like you are losing friends or protection. You may find you miss the extra attention you received during treatment. Some patients even feel "let down" after being stressed so long about getting through treatment.

The family and friends who were there to support you during treatment may not be around as much, or as supportive, when treatment ends. Suddenly, you may feel like you are facing the future alone. It may be hard for you to explain to others your ambivalent feelings about the end of treatment, especially when people tend to view your survival after treatment as the end of the road. They may not fully appreciate that you can't simply shed the role of "patient" overnight.

Aftereffects of Treatment

Chances are that you will have some physical and emotional effects after treatment. Some of these effects will subside soon after treatment ends, while others may fade slowly over months or even years. You may experience chronic pain or difficulties due to treatment-related side effects. You may even be facing permanent loss of a limb or an organ, or other significant changes in your body's appearance or functioning. Learning to adapt to these changes in your body can be challenging.

Fatigue is the most common side effect of cancer and its treatment. The extent of your fatigue will depend on the type of cancer and treatment that you received, but you may find yourself feeling run down for some time after treatment is completed. There are several factors that can contribute to fatigue, such as a low red blood cell count, hormonal changes, and the energy requirements your body needs to recover. Psychological factors can also contribute significantly to fatigue. If your lack of energy is accompanied by other symptoms, such as clinical depression, you should seek help from a professional in psychosocial services (see Chapter 3).

The changes that cancer has caused to your body and to your life can bring about other powerful emotions. You now have the "luxury" of being aware of negative feelings, now that you are no longer caught in a whirlwind of hospital visits. You may find yourself angry about the unfairness of getting cancer and about what you've been through. You may also be angry and disappointed at family and friends who did not support you through treatment. Anger and frustration can also result from dealing with the physical changes caused by treatment, and the lingering effects that the disease and treatment have had on your family's well being. Anger is a good sign—it shows you still have a lot of fight left in you. You can recognize and express these feelings in healthy ways (see Chapter 2). At the same time, you can make some choices to use your anger as energy for healing yourself and your family.

Fear of Recurrence

Once you have had cancer, there is always the possibility of recurrence, although with many types of cancer, recurrence is less likely. For most people with cancer, the chance their cancer may come back is one of the hardest issues to deal with after treatment ends. The thought of your cancer coming back can be upsetting. Many patients ignore any little "voices of doubt" they feel. This can only make it worse. The healthy approach is to know that it is normal to worry. As you face this fear, it usually lessens over time. The coping skills that you have used throughout your cancer experience will be helpful in dealing with your concerns about recurrence. You may need to put some of your worries to rest by taking action, such as facing bills that may have accumulated. However, if you often think about recurrence and feel so scared that you cannot function in your usual role, or if you feel stuck, you may want to talk to a mental health professional (see Chapter 3).

Because of the possibility of recurrence, it may be most accurate to think of cancer as a chronic disease that needs to be monitored and cared for throughout your life, rather than a one-time illness that can be cured by a short period of treatment. You will probably feel a great deal of anxiety prior to visits to your doctor and follow-up tests, such as CT scans and MRIs, but remember that these visits represent close monitoring of your health. And with each successful visit to your doctor, you'll probably become more reassured about your health.

Questions to Ask Your Doctor About Follow-Up Care

You may want to ask the following questions about follow-up care:

- Which of my medical team members is in charge of my follow-up care?
- How often will I have follow-up examinations?
- What blood work, x-rays, or other tests will I undergo during these exams?
- How long will I have to undergo follow-up care?
- What are symptoms that I should watch out for?
- Who can best answer my questions and concerns?
- Will my follow-up care be covered by my insurance?

☙

What Your Children May Be Feeling Now That Treatment Is Over

Like you, your children have had to face their fears and make adjustments during diagnosis and treatment of your cancer. Now that your treatment is over, they may resist making adjustments again, or they may have trouble understanding why things can't simply go back to the way they were before. Your children may also be dealing with fears that your cancer will come back, or they may be angry with the way things have changed. They may have trouble identifying these negative feelings, or they may express them in unhealthy ways. Children are flexible, adaptive creatures, but the time after treatment can nonetheless be a bumpy ride for the whole family.

Your children may be troubled by the change they have had to weather over a relatively short period of time, during your diagnosis, treatment, and now, recovery. They have witnessed intense emotions in their parents that they may not have seen before. They have experienced changes in their daily routines, and have been getting less attention. If the parent with cancer is their primary caretaker, they may have had someone new, perhaps with a different style, taking care of them. Maybe the house has been renovated to accommodate the changes in your health, or the family diet has been altered.

All of these changes may leave children feeling that the world is unpredictable, which can make them feel insecure, afraid, or angry. They may even misbehave. It will help your children if you acknowledge that it is normal for them to be upset about all of the changes. At the same time, you will have to be straightforward with your children about the things that cannot go back to the way they used to be. Share how long it may take for you to get over lingering effects of treatment, such as fatigue. Your children will find it reassuring if you and your family can establish a routine after treatment ends. By providing structure, safety, and support in every area where possible, you can help your children to see the world as stable and predictable.

Children's Fears of Recurrence

Like you, your children may be afraid that your cancer will return. They may be quite open about their fears. They may even ask you repeatedly about the

Children's Common Reactions After Treatment

Your children may

- Have a hard time understanding why you are not immediately 100% well after your treatment and why things can't go back to the way they used to be.
- Cling to you and resent any demands on your time.
- Be afraid that you will get sick again and they will lose your attention to the disease once more.
- Have become withdrawn during your treatment, and may be slow to warm up and get close to you again.
- Be reluctant to talk about their fears that your cancer may come back.
- Irrationally believe that just by talking about your sickness, they may bring it back.
- Be on high alert for any signs that something is wrong again.
- Misinterpret a headache or a stomachache, or may worry unnecessarily about your checkups, especially if they sense your own anxiety.

Your teenager(s) may

- Have gained a feeling of independence during your treatment, because there was less attention focused on them, and they may resent any renewed infringements on their freedom.

These behaviors and feelings will likely pass with time, but it will also help for you to talk with your children about what they're thinking and feeling, and to use the hands-on tools at the end of this chapter with your family.

෨෬

possibility of recurrence. On the other hand, they may keep their fears bottled-up inside, or have trouble putting them into words. They may sense your anxiety before check-ups, and may come to their own conclusions regarding why you are going to the doctor again.

The best policy is to be completely honest and straightforward with your children about the possibility of recurrence. This is needed even if you are tempted to protect them from this hard fact. They will be much better prepared to cope, should your cancer return. By approaching this subject with them, it encourages them to talk about their concerns and to ask questions. Praise your children for sharing their feelings. When they ask about recurrence, explain to them the symptoms that you will be looking for. Reassure them that you will let them know about any developments, but that you expect all to go well. You can help them develop a realistic perspective by telling them that some people die from cancer, but a lot of people get better and live to be very old. You may also want to stress to them that you have gotten through treatment once before, and you will do it again if you have to.

Teenagers Can Present Special Challenges After Treatment

Your teenagers were already going through a turbulent time in their life when cancer came along. They are at a developmental stage where they are beginning to separate from their parents and define who they are as adults. They may find it difficult to cope with the time after treatment. They may feel like they are being forced back into the family just as they were beginning to break free and gain their independence. They may also have lost some of their privacy because of changes made to your home to accommodate your recovery. The normal acts of rebellion that may occur at this time can be hurtful to you. You may feel they blame you for having had cancer, but chances are this behavior is a normal part of growing up. However, as with during your diagnosis and treatment, it is still important that you set limits and maintain discipline to let adolescents know that Mom and Dad are still in control.

Working through the activities at the end of this chapter can help you and your children overcome the fears and other negative emotions that are normal after undergoing cancer treatment. However, you should watch for more serious signs of trouble in your children that may require the intervention of a professional. If your children or teenagers are showing significant behavior changes, such as changes in eating or sleeping habits, school problems, fear, anxiety, depression, or suicidal thoughts, seek help from a counseling professional as soon as possible (see Chapter 3).

How You and Your Family Can Thrive After Treatment

Cancer has probably put you and your family through some pretty tough times by now. However, people who have survived cancer find that they reevaluate their lives and their priorities, and discover the strength and unity of their families. Each day becomes a precious gift. You can learn to explore how you and your family can move beyond cancer and enjoy together this new appreciation for life.

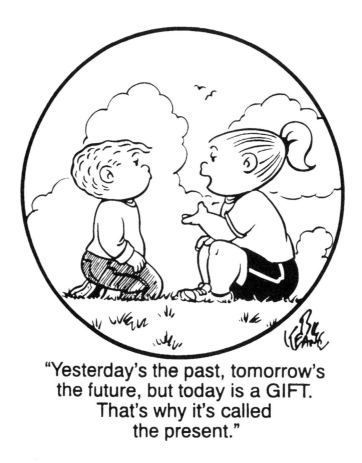

"Yesterday's the past, tomorrow's
the future, but today is a GIFT.
That's why it's called
the present."

Reprinted with special permission of King Features Syndicate. © 1999 B.T. Keane, Inc.

Survivor's Tips for Life After Treatment

These are tidbits of wisdom gathered from survivors over the years:

- Take life one day at a time, and make sure to cherish everything around you.
- Be kind to yourself.
- Help others. Reaching out to someone else can reduce the stress caused by brooding.
- Learn to pace yourself, and to take a break before you get too tired.
- Get enough exercise. It's a great way to get rid of tension and anger in a positive way.
- Eat properly and get enough sleep.
- Let your loved ones know how much they mean to you. Tell all the people who have supported you during your battle with cancer how much their thoughtfulness and caring have helped you. This will make you feel better too.
- Smell the roses—you've made it through treatment! Now's the time to reassess what is truly special in your life.
- Reward yourself. Celebrate! Do something special just for you. Get a massage or take a walk in beautiful surroundings, or use some quiet time to relax.

ᏛᎧ

What You Need Now

Now that your treatment is over, chances are you need some time to yourself, to reclaim your well being, and to think about where you are now in life, and where you are going. You will need time to take care of yourself physically, by getting exercise and going to your follow-up appointments. Sometimes you may feel guilty that these activities take time away from your spouse and children. But, keep in mind that taking care of yourself benefits the whole family. It's not the quantity of time you spend with your family that matters, it's the quality of your time together. In addition, by healing yourself emotionally, you will also teach your children about coping and healing.

Don't be afraid to ask your family for what you need now to get better. You will need to ease into activities gradually. Due to lingering fatigue, your energies are probably still very limited. Arrange for breaks from the children and your household responsibilities. Let your family and friends know how much their continued support will help you as you slowly regain your life and your daily routines.

Managing Your Feelings

People who have survived cancer commonly report that the time after treatment was the most difficult for them emotionally. You, too, are probably now going through some turbulent feelings. Prepare yourself to be vulnerable to strong emotions at follow-up visits, anniversary dates of your diagnosis, or television movies about cancer. Anything that reminds you of your experience can make you feel sad, anxious, or angry. As you weather these emotions, healing occurs from the inside out. Scars (emotional and physical) may remain, but the pain will subside. The painful emotions that you may be feeling now will heal as time passes. It is also very important that you forgive yourself for having powerful emotions now. You may be tempted to chide yourself—isn't it time you got over this? But when you were in the midst of battling cancer, you probably didn't have much time or energy to explore your emotions. It's understandable if your negative feelings about what you have been through are just now catching up with you.

There are some things you can do, though, to help you manage these feelings. The techniques for taking care of yourself during treatment that you learned about in Chapter 4, such as journal keeping, relaxation exercises, and cognitive techniques, can also help you now. Try some activities that might help you to focus outside yourself, such as volunteering or taking a class. If, however, you find your emotions still out of control despite taking these steps, do not hesitate to seek help from a counseling professional. You may especially need outside help if, for example, you find you're taking your anger out on your family, or if you are experiencing any of the warning signs of depression (see Chapter 3).

Seeking Support

If you feel isolated because of your experiences, or want to better understand what you are going through now, consider joining a cancer survivor's support group (see Chapter 3). Ask yourself if such a group is right for you. Are you comfortable sharing your feelings with others who have been through a similar situation? Are you interested in hearing about the experiences other cancer survivors have had, and the feelings they are dealing with? Could you benefit from their advice? While your family has no doubt been sympathetic, fellow cancer survivors can truly identify with what you have been going through.

If you feel that a support group is not a good option for you, or if you want to supplement your support group experience, there are many other resources available that can help. For example, there are many books, tapes, newsletters, magazines, telephone resources, and organizations that can help (see Resource Guide). The Internet has become one of the fastest growing sources of information and support for people with cancer, and it is important that you visit reputable sites. One such site is the American Cancer Society's Cancer Survivor's Network (www.acscsn.org), which offers a community for cancer survivors, families, and friends to share experiences.

You also may find it emotionally satisfying to reach out to others who are now struggling with cancer. You no doubt have helpful insights on getting through diagnosis and treatment. You may also now want to "give back" to the cancer community in other ways. You might, for example, become involved in cancer prevention and treatment as a cause. You could support your local hospital cancer unit through fund-raising activities. Helping with the fight against cancer in these ways can become a part of your healing process.

Helping Your Children Adjust and Thrive

There are several things you can do to help your children now that you and your family have reached this point. One important element to helping your children adapt and thrive now is to re-establish a family routine. It may not be the same routine as before. Although, it will help if you can bring back habits and traditions that are important to you and your family. The important thing is to provide structure and support in every area possible, such as having dinner or bedtime at the same time every day. Establishing a routine again can help your children to see the world as stable and predictable, which can help them to feel secure.

Family Meetings

If you haven't already done so, now may be a good time to start having family meetings (see Chapter 2). These meetings can help your children feel their input is valued and that they are being kept "in the know." Getting the family together on a regular basis can help air out tensions before they get too high, and to talk about what everyone needs now. For example, are your children feeling like they want more togetherness? Or perhaps more independence? When addressing problems like this at a family meeting, be sure to focus on workable, practical solutions, rather than just letting complaints take over the meeting.

Getting your family together for meetings also gives you a chance to keep everyone informed about how your priorities have changed, and what the plans are as you look forward. Your career goals may totally change, for example. As a result of your experiences with cancer, you might find that the work you're doing is not meaningful to you and decide to go back to school. Your whole family will be affected by decisions like this because of the impact they will have on the family income and on the time you have to spend with your family. But keeping everyone advised of these developments at an early stage will help everyone adjust to your plans as they take shape.

Family meetings are best for information sharing, reassurance, and making plans. These meetings, however, are probably not a good time to explore everyone's emotions. Your children are more likely to share their feelings during one-on-one time with you and your spouse.

Make Private Time for Each Child

Be sure to set aside private time for each of your children on a regular basis. You can use this time together to do fun, relaxed activities, or just to talk. Spending time with each child will help them feel loved and cherished. It's also a good time for you to help your children express themselves and share what they're feeling now with you. Getting children to expose their feelings can be hard at times, in part because they themselves may not be "tuned in" to what they're feeling. Try asking open questions to help them get at what they're feeling, such as "What scares you most, now that my treatment is over?" You might also try probing for more specific information by asking more targeted questions, such as "How does it make you feel when I go for my check-ups?" or "How does it make you feel when I can't tuck you in because I'm at my support group meeting?" Be sure to praise your children when they do open up to you, and let them know that it's normal to feel bad, even after treatment is over. There are also some ways to help your children with specific emotions they may be coping with now, such as sadness or anger.

If Your Children Are Sad

Of all the emotions your children may be coping with now, sadness may be the one that is most difficult to examine or put into words. Children may be grieving specific losses, such as the times they could not be with you while you were sick, or the important recital that you were unable to attend. Their sadness might also be due to something more abstract or indefinable. Examples of this may be the loss of innocence or the discovery that the world is not such a safe place after all. Rather than trying to explore their sadness rationally, the best thing you can do for children who are grieving is offer them simple physical comfort and soothing words. Give your children permission to grieve, too. By cuddling and comforting your children, and by letting them know it's okay to feel sad, you can give them a safe and secure place to work through their sorrow and adjust to their losses.

If Your Children Are Worried or Afraid

If your children express feelings of fear or anxiety, try to probe further to find out what they are afraid of so you will know how to reassure them. It's quite likely that your children are afraid your cancer will come back, especially if they pick up on the anxiety you may be feeling before each follow-up visit. Be straightforward with your children about the possibility of recurrence, and reassure them that you will let them know about any changes in your health status. Talk to them about how check-ups make you feel. You can let them know that check-ups make you afraid too, but that this doesn't mean anything bad is going to happen. This will help keep them from jumping to their own terrible conclusions about why you're going to the doctor again.

You can explain that worrying about the future is normal, but help them to set limits on their worrying. You can let them know it's okay to ask you about the possibility of recurrence, but urge them to live as though everything is going to work out. Equipping your children to live with uncertainty will not only help them now, it's a skill they can use for the rest of their lives. You can use examples from your children's day-to-day lives to show them how worrying didn't make a difference, but only made them spend more time feeling bad. Point out that the time spent worrying is a loss. Then you might discuss a time they made a back-up plan which helped them put their worries aside. Encourage your children to determine what they can do for now to ease their worries. Finally, assure your children that even if your cancer does return, their needs will be met.

If Your Children Are Angry

You may find your children expressing anger or frustration at times. They may throw tantrums, slam doors, or lash out at siblings. Discuss any observed tensions or resentment, and try to determine what is making your children angry by asking them targeted questions. Ask them, for example, if they blame you for getting sick. Or is it that they think things should be back to normal by now? Are they frustrated that you still don't have so much time to spend with them, or you're too fatigued to go to the park?

Once you have gotten a better sense of what is making your children angry, praise them for sharing their feelings, and let them know it's normal to feel mad after treatment is over. Acknowledge their losses, whether they seem significant or not. For example, you might say, "I know you haven't been able to go to soccer practice since I've been sick" or "I know I missed your school play last month," and acknowledge that you know it's been hard for them. If

Helping Children Thrive After Treatment

- Set aside private time for each of your children. Make it special, a ritual that only you and your child share, like reading in bed, playing cards, or drawing pictures together.
- Let your children know that you're available for them, anytime they need to talk about anything that's on their mind.
- Find out if there's a support group for children whose parents have had cancer that your children can attend.
- Give your children hugs or back rubs. Physical comfort can express volumes to your children about how loved, cherished, and secure they are.
- Have fun too! Do something you've all always wanted to do like going to a theme park or flying a kite. Play a fun board game. Have a water fight in the backyard!

ନ୍ତେ

talking about what is making your children angry doesn't help, you might try encouraging them to vent their feelings in other ways (see Chapter 2, page 51). For example, any activity that expends energy without hurting anyone or anything may help. You might have your children kick a soccer ball around (but not in the house), or draw a picture of what is making them mad—then tear it up into many pieces. Encourage your children to punch pillows. You could even punch pillows with them. Who knows, you might all end up in a pile on the floor, covered with pillows, giggling helplessly, and forgetting, at least for a little while, about all your worldly concerns! The point is that indulging in a little silliness will go a long way in helping your children release their anger and learn other ways of coping.

Hands-On Tools

The time after treatment is a good time to process what has taken place over the past several months. These activities may help bring closure for you and your children. Not all of the exercises will be right for your children. As with the other exercises, feel free to adapt them to what will work best for your family.

◆   *Create a "healing space" in your house* that helps to recognize that healing continues even after treatment is over. In this place, you might ask every family member to find and leave a symbol of healing. For example, a stone might be for strength (because it's rock hard). You might place a family picture or a picture of yourself. Place an empty pill bottle or other object that would suggest being sick in the space. You and your children may want to add some objects for their beauty such as fall leaves. Children might bring things home from school or from a walk in the yard. Looking at this place can help you and your children center and focus on being relaxed. You can add objects to your healing place at any time, so that it becomes an ongoing project.

◆   *Help your children make a video* about what the experience has been like for them. Or, suggest that they perform a play to show how they felt throughout treatment. You can see how they "play" you and relate to you and each other.

◆   *Have your children draw or construct a see-saw structure* on a piece of posterboard. Use a paper fastener so that it has moveable parts. You can use "blocks" made out of paper and attach them to the arms of the see-saw with velcro. They can be added to a drawn-on see-saw with masking tape. This activity shows how we need support to balance ourselves and our families.

◆ *Write a special saying* on a large piece of posterboard with a magic marker in large letters. Then cut the board into several pieces and have your children put the pieces together. You can also purchase blank puzzles at hobby or craft stores.

◆ *Have your children draw a cartoon strip* describing your illness, from the time of diagnosis to now when treatment has been completed. They could each work on a separate "frame" for the story.

◆ *Play charades with your children* to help demonstrate feelings. Give them a charade card and ask them to act out the emotion on the card or describe each situation to your children and ask them how they would act it out.

◆ *Draw a target on a large piece of paper* and explain to your children that the circles represent our support systems. The small dot in the middle represents you. The inner circle represents those close to you who support you and who feel closest to you. The next circle is for people who you are not the closest to, but those who you can go to for support or who have given you support (e.g., co-workers, church, school, and organizations). The last circle is used to identify broader forms of support. They are those agencies, groups, etc. that you know are there if you need them. Have everyone fill out their own circles, and follow up with a good discussion. This can be a way to remind everyone of all the support they have found along the way that will always be there for them.

CHAPTER SIX

Helping Children
deal with recurrence,
progressive, or terminal illness

M any of the same issues you faced after your initial diagnosis will surface again if your illness has returned. The difference now, of course, is that you will probably be more worried than you might have been in the beginning. Depending on the kind of cancer you have, it could even be many years since your initial diagnosis and you may have forgotten much of what you went through. If it has not been very long since your initial diagnosis, the feelings of fear and uncertainty will be fresh in your mind and difficult to deal with again so soon.

It may seem impossible to start over again. All of a sudden, life feels chaotic and survival less than certain. It is important to remember that you don't need to be perfect and that you are your children's best source of security. Your love for them is one of the most important factors in how they will manage, so try to be realistic in terms of what you expect of yourself. You may need to rely on the help of others again for some period of time during active treatment. While it can be difficult to ask for help, usually it's only temporary until you are feeling more in control.

What You May Be Facing

What you may experience now are feelings of sadness and grief as your life is turned upside down again. What was certain about life is no longer certain. You may go through a period of depression and grieve the loss of the normalcy of life. Parents often describe a feeling of betrayal. They say things like, "I did everything that was recommended (surgery, chemotherapy, or radiation) and the cancer still came back."

You also may feel insecure about your financial situation as your medical expenses continue to rise. You may worry about your job security and how you will be able to pay all of the bills. If you felt like you could barely make ends meet before, you may feel a heavy burden and sense of dread about impending debt.

Feelings of anger, fear, and anxiety will surface again, maybe greater than before, and you may feel much more vulnerable than when you were first diagnosed. That is to be expected. It will be important to manage your fears so that you can use your energy for dealing with recurrent disease. If you are having trouble doing that, you might want to consider getting psychosocial help (see Chapter 3).

You may be afraid that your situation is hopeless. In general, that is not the case, but much depends on the kind of cancer you have and your response to treatment. Before the past fifty years, there was little to be done once a cancer had recurred. This is no longer true since there have been so many advances in treatment and the management of its side effects. Certainly, the situation is more serious if the cancer has returned, but for many patients, it means that treatment now will be more intense than the first treatment.

You may be wondering if it is worthwhile to go through more treatment. This reaction is often the result of feelings of panic and desperation rather than the medical reality. There are often more options to consider and making a decision may seem overwhelming. Since every patient responds differently to treatment, you need to make sure you think through all of your options. You should fully explore the advances made in cancer treatment. Based on your doctor's recommendation and feedback from your family, you should decide what is right for you. If you are uncertain about what to do next, it may be useful to consider a second opinion from a doctor at another facility (e.g., a comprehensive cancer center or university teaching hospital). This is important because you will want to be sure that you fully understand your options and carefully weigh the cost and benefits to your quality of life.

Things to Consider if Cancer Has Spread to Many Areas

When cancer spreads to many areas of the body, treatment decisions become more complicated. Your choices depend a great deal on your understanding of your disease, your trust in your health care team, as well as your and your family's well being. In general, an untreated cancer is more difficult to deal with than if you are doing something to control its growth. Your doctor should be able to explain to you the pros and cons of continued treatment and help you decide which course will meet your needs, both medically and emotionally. For some people, doing nothing is impossible, and for others, quality of life becomes the chief concern.

Whatever you decide in terms of how long to go on with aggressive cancer treatment, you should know that "supportive care" is always an option. This means it will be important to deal with the symptoms of the disease even if your focus shifts away from expecting to be cured. For example, there are medicines to control nausea and relieve pain. Fatigue and your quality of life can be markedly different if you are taking advantage of the most up-to-date methods of controlling side effects. Be sure you have an accurate picture of all that is available in the management of advanced disease.

If you are having trouble getting or sorting out information, you can call the American Cancer Society at any time. If you need to discuss your family situation in more depth, find out if your treatment center is staffed with oncology social workers or other mental health professionals. These people know a great deal about solving family problems related to cancer and can help you sort out your options and deal with your family.

Explaining Recurrence to Children

Because there can be so many management options for cancer that has spread from the original site, you may be facing many more months of treatment and will need to make a plan as to how you and your family can best manage this.

It will be almost impossible to conceal the reality of cancer. **Children who have not been told the truth about a parent's illness will have a much harder time coping.** By "telling the truth", we mean what the child needs to know in terms of what is going on with his or her life. Children do not need to know every thought or worry that you have, only enough to manage their own fears and continue to function in school, with their peers, and with as much security as you can build into their lives.

Reflect on what your children were told about your illness. Building on that information, you can go on to say that the cancer has now come back. Tell the children you will need to be treated again with stronger medicines or radiation treatments, depending on the treatment plan. It may be useful to review basic cancer terms (see Chapter 2). Children often misunderstand the meaning of the new or unfamiliar. Do not assume too much in terms of how they understand what they are told. For example, one child insisted that his mother's cancer had gone away because her hair was growing back after her course of chemotherapy. It can be useful to ask your children to tell you what they know about the situation so you can correct the things they do not understand.

As discussed earlier, children will need to know how your treatment will affect their lives. They need to know what side effects are likely to happen, what changes in the family routine will need to be made, and when they can expect life to return to normal. You may feel very sad and unsettled that your children have to go through this upheaval again. It is no one's fault the cancer has come back, and you can only do your best to help them adjust to the changes which may need to be made in family life as a result. Starting treatment again may make the family feel very unsettled. It's important to acknowledge this, but try to be matter-of-fact about it rather than apologetic. There are ways to manage this family crisis. You will need everyone's suggestions about how family members can adjust to temporary changes in the family's routines.

Weekly family meetings may be a good way to stay in touch with what's going on with everyone. You might tell your children that this is a special time reserved for the family members to talk about anything that is bothering them. You can also use the activities at the end of this chapter to help your children talk about things that are important. If you are expecting a difficult week ahead, you can prepare them by talking about what will be done to keep life as normal as possible. Let them know that you may not be able to help with activities like homework, car pools, and softball practice. Explain that you will need to make other plans so their routines can continue, with other people filling in until you are feeling better.

The family schedule may need to be changed to fit an intensive treatment plan. You may need to do more low-key activities so you are not taxing your resources. Think of low-energy activities that allow you to still be together such as watching television, reading a book, or playing a board game. The message here is that you are still in charge of what is going on in their lives and they are not on their own.

Understanding Children's Reactions to Recurrence

In order to evaluate how your children might react to the progression of cancer, you will need to consider their ages, their personalities, and their relationships with you and extended family members. You know your children better than anyone, so you can probably predict how they will behave when facing this added stress in the family. Remember that your children are individuals and what works for one may not work for another.

The stages your children are at in their development will be important in understanding their reactions to progressive disease. For young children, there will obviously be more need for actual caretaking. You might need to call on other family members or friends if energy is low. Younger children have more of a tendency to regress and lose ground in what they have learned to do for themselves. They are also less able to express how they feel in words. A child who has just become toilet trained may start having accidents. Another child who has made a good adjustment to school might start having problems separating from a parent again. Children with learning disabilities might have more problems paying attention than before. While these behaviors usually get better once the situation stabilizes, other family members or friends might be called upon to give your younger children more attention.

Teenagers may be a big challenge. They are struggling with becoming more independent and can appear more distant or detached from the life of the family. Because teens often have trouble talking with their parents, you may need to make a special effort to reach them. Feelings of worry, anger, or even resentment may get in the way of their sharing. Try to arrange a special time for teenagers, separate from your other children.

One of the issues for teens is that they can realistically assume more responsibility around the house during times when a parent might be especially ill or tired. Sometimes older children are depended upon too much and resentments build up. It will be important to help find a balance between home and outside responsibilities. Let your teenagers know that you realize that maintaining school activities and their relationships with friends is still important (see Chapter 2).

The behaviors that children use to express their worries about progressive cancer can really tax a parent's reserves. That's why it is especially important to ask for help from other family or friends. If that is not possible, talk to the staff where you are being treated about community support services (see Chapter 3).

Dealing with Uncertainty and Anxiety

Some of the questions that children have now will be the same as those after diagnosis. But, now the situation is more serious since the disease has progressed. The most obvious worry children have is what will happen to them if their parent should die. Depending on their age, the "who will take care of me?" question is the most critical. This is also the one that is the hardest for children to ask because they fear the answer. The fear of being left alone is one of our greatest fears and children with a chronically ill parent may feel this quite strongly. Handling this is probably one of the most painful experiences a parent might have. You might have discussed this in a general way when you were first diagnosed. Now, if your cancer is progressing, you will need to address it more directly.

Obviously, this is a very difficult situation, but you and your family still need to find ways to go on. Many parents find that living with uncertainty is the most difficult part of having cancer. Since no one can really predict the future, the challenge is to find a way to deal with day-to-day living. One way you can help is to find something positive in the situation. For instance, if you are feeling exhausted from daily radiation treatments, you might enlist the help of a favorite aunt who could take your children to the zoo. Or, you can give them something to look forward to, such as going to the movies. Finding something good in the situation is a better way of coping than living with "doom and gloom" most of the time. It is good for you and your children to have some "time-outs." It's not productive to focus on the worst possible outcome all of the time.

People differ in the way they see the world. There are some people who are naturally optimistic and others who see black clouds most of the time. While there is nothing good about the possibility that a parent might die, finding meaning in the experience can be very valuable. Asking yourself and your children what you have learned or gained from all that's happened helps give some meaning to your experience. Thinking through and asking your children what meaning they have found may lead to special insights. The proverb, "a joy shared is multiplied and a grief shared is divided", is very applicable to your life right now. Sharing these thoughts and feelings can allow you to see incredible strengths in yourself and your children. If it's the mother in the family who is sick, the children might become closer to Dad. Helping your children see how they cope with adversity builds inner strength for now and future life stresses. While this is something we wish children might never have to endure, it will serve them well to learn how to cope with life's challenges.

Children react to reality as they experience it around them. For instance, if many family members have died from cancer, a child might assume that a person with cancer always dies. Or, if a parent looks the same as they always did, it may never occur to them that death is a possibility. So encourage your children to tell you what they think might happen as in, "What worries do you have about the treatment and my cancer? What thoughts do you have about the treatment not working?" This way, you have some sense about your children's understanding of the situation. Depending on your understanding of your prognosis, you might say something like, "Some people with a recurrence of cancer still get better. I'm going to do all that I can to make it. I'll tell you if the treatment has stopped working." The point is to reassure your children that you have made provisions for their welfare if the worst should happen.

Facing Questions About Death and the Future

How Adults Deal with Death

Some people deal with death by asking the question, "Why me?" Trying to make sense of it all and searching for the answer can cause many sleepless nights and incredible soul searching. Some people find that it doesn't really matter why something has happened, they just want to know how to deal with it. Many people initially think that if only they know why something has happened— if they *do* or *stop doing* something—that somehow the situation will change. While this notion is not necessarily rational, it illustrates the way people think. We all look for reasons for what happens in our lives. It is hard to accept that cancer can be a totally random event and that there may be no answer to why a person has gotten the disease and may die. There are many forces that can influence the development of cancer. These can be genetic, environmental, or related to behavior such as smoking. A person may never know why they have cancer so trying to find the answer to this question only produces frustration and drains the parent of energy needed to cope with reality.

For some people, the answer to the "why me" question is something they could have influenced like the link between cigarette smoking and lung cancer. These patients can have a much harder time coping with cancer because they feel guilty that something they did could have caused their cancer. The job for them is to forgive themselves. If they cannot do this and focus on dealing with the here and now, coping is usually much harder. Many times it helps to talk to an oncology social worker or cancer counselor to make peace with this issue.

The bottom line in addressing the "why me" question is that knowing the answer to the question will not change the course of the illness. While the question usually cannot be answered, if you remain focused on the question, it will interfere with how well you are able to cope. Worrying about "why" will drain your energy. Rather than ask why, it is better to reflect on the meaning of the illness to you. That energy is better used in dealing with the reality of helping yourself and your family deal with a chronic illness. Consider getting some counseling if you find yourself unable to move away from this issue (see Chapter 3).

What to Tell Your Children

What you tell your children about death depends on your understanding of the nature of your illness and how treatment will impact your future. For instance, there are some cancers which progress at a fairly slow pace and treatment can be expected, if not to cure, then to control its growth for some time. There are other cancers that are more difficult to manage, and plans for the future need to be made. In that case, the parent may play out for the child the worst possible scenario as a way of taming the fears a child will be experiencing. A parent might say something like, "In case you're worrying about what will happen if the treatment doesn't work and I'm not around, I've already talked this over with Aunt Susie and she will be here for you." Or, a mother might say, "If Dad doesn't make it, I'll need to go back to work but I will still be here to take care of you."

Regardless of prognosis, all people with cancer need to learn how to manage the uncertainty of living with cancer. The best a parent can do is to acknowledge the possibility of death while focusing on living each day. Many people with cancer say that once they acknowledge this, they are better able to get on with life. Parents need to focus on hope for the future unless it becomes certain death is inevitable. Even then, there will be a future for your children. As hard as it might seem, children can grieve for the loss of a parent and find a way to go on with their lives. Keep in mind that you have already had a positive influence on who they will be as adults and that will not disappear if you are not physically present to see them into adulthood.

If it looks like treatment is not working and the possibility is that you may not survive, children should be told that the cancer has come back. Children need to know what you have decided about treatment or supportive care. If you want more treatment, you might say, "The doctors will need to try stronger medicines to try to get my cancer under control again." You should say that it is possible that this will not work, but that you and the doctor will be trying very hard to prevent that from happening. Again, tell your children that you will be honest with them if it looks like you will not survive. This may be extremely difficult or impossible for you to do. This is very understandable, and if so, your spouse or partner may be the one to have this conversation.

In single parent families, perhaps another close relative or friend can be called upon (see Chapter 7). If that is not possible, someone on the health care team may be called upon to talk to the children. This could be an oncology social worker, nurse, or the doctor, but someone needs to communicate to the children the possibility that a parent might not survive. If this is not done, children can feel very angry for years afterward that they were not prepared for a parent's death. Obviously, this information should only be communicated if there is no doubt that the parent will not survive.

What You Can Say

If death is a possibility, you can address the topic in such a way that is realistic but will not make your children unbearably anxious. These are examples of what you might say:

- Some people with cancer get all better and some don't. I am trying my best to get better.
- You know this is a serious situation. It's possible that I could die but I'm not doing that right now so let's focus on living.
- I'm not sure how I will do. It all depends on how I respond to treatment—let's give the chemotherapy (or radiation) another chance to work.

Providing children with balanced responses will help them cope. Even if you know for sure that death will probably occur at some point, your family will need a way to go on living. And so will you. There is no way people can live anything close to a normal life if they are totally focused on the future and how it might be if the worst happens. If death is a possibility, it should be acknowledged as such, but put into the perspective that life has to go on until death is imminent.

Testing Faith

For some families, a strong faith is very helpful in getting through cancer treatment, and this faith will be a source of continuing comfort when the going gets rough. For others, this experience will really test their faith and they may find themselves questioning God or some higher power in ways they have never experienced.

Your children may also be struggling with the question of how a higher power could allow their parent to have cancer or die. The way you deal with this has everything to do with how you as the parent answer this question for yourself. The issue of "why bad things happen to good people" is a struggle for most human beings. Do you believe that God chooses which people will get cancer, perhaps as some sort of punishment for past mistakes? Or is cancer more of a random event, which God allows to happen? Some people may even be unsure that there is a Supreme Being and will bring that uncertainty to the cancer experience. No one can answer this profound question for someone else because the answer relates to who you are as a person, your upbringing, and your overall philosophy of life. It is not unusual for people with cancer to go through periods when they really question their faith or feel that they may be losing their faith. If this is the case, you may receive some comfort from talking this over with a spiritual advisor or with someone who is comfortable dealing with spiritual issues.

What Children Understand About Death

Infants do not have a concept of death, but are aware of a parent's absence.

Toddlers feel anxious when someone is sick, and they confuse death with sleep. For example, when a young girl found her bird dead in the cage, she thought he was sleeping. Her father gently told her that the bird was dead, and she said, "Well, when is he not going to be dead?"

Preschoolers understand that people die, but they are unable to understand that death is final. They think that death is temporary and can be reversed. They may believe their own thoughts can cause a person's illness or death.

School-Agers view death as final and frightening. They also develop curiosity about death.

Teenagers understand that death can happen to anyone at any age. They have an adult understanding of death.

இஇ

It is not necessary for you to have all of the answers in order to help your children with this issue. You should address these questions within the context of what you believe and what you have taught your children to believe about how religion impacts people's lives. For instance, if you believe in a merciful being rather than a vengeful one, you may want to tell your children that your family is not being punished. If you are not sure where a higher being fits into your life, it's okay to share that uncertainty. You can say something like, "I'm not really sure at this point how I feel about God. Some days I'm really angry and not sure what to believe." The point is to be truthful and consistent in terms of how you have dealt with the question of religion in the past. If you try to comfort your children with a belief system that you're not really sure of, they will probably pick up on this and be more confused.

The important thing will be to give your children an opportunity to express how they are feeling. This may be a tough area to address if you are feeling uncertain yourself about how to make peace with what has happened to you and your family. It's okay to say that you don't know where to put God into the picture. You should let them know that most people go through periods when they feel angry that God has allowed this to happen. Anger is a difficult emotion for many people. But, your children will benefit from knowing that expressing angry feelings may make them feel better in the end rather than stifling how they feel about your illness. This may feel very scary to you, but usually their anger is about the situation, not about you.

Some people find that the whole question of their relationship to a higher power is shaken as a result of having cancer. If this is so, you may want to pay some attention to this and seek help from someone who is comfortable with these issues. There may be times when friends or relatives try to reassure you with comments like "God doesn't give us anything we can't handle," or "God must have a reason that this has happened." People say these things with the very best of intentions. If you are struggling with spiritual doubts, such comments might only increase the amount of stress you're feeling. It will be even harder then to help your children find a way to make sense out of what is going on. Talking with a pastoral counselor might offer a safe place to come to terms with what you believe for yourself. If you are not already connected to a church or faith group and need a spiritual counselor, ask your health care team for a referral (see Chapter 3).

Understanding Children's Reactions to a Parent's Potential Death

Children's reactions to the possibility of a parent's death depend on many things. Some factors include the child's personality, relationship to the sick parent, age, and development, along with how imminent or distant the death is thought to be. Some children will refuse to believe that their parent is sick and will show this in their behavior. For instance, they may become whiney and irritable, and act out their feelings by refusing to go along with what they know to be the family rules. Sometimes children will withdraw from others in their family. They may even refuse to listen to an explanation of what is going on or pretend that nothing is wrong. They may behave badly and act out their confusion and anxiety. For example, children may resist going to school, or pick fights with a favorite sibling. These behaviors will be very upsetting to parents who will probably not have as much energy as usual to cope with their children.

Anger is probably the most common reaction that people have to the stress related to a serious illness. Anger is also one of the more difficult issues to deal with because many people have a hard time expressing that emotion directly. Many of us have been taught that it is not acceptable to be angry, so these feelings get stifled. Then, when we face a situation like cancer where anger is normal, we do not feel comfortable expressing the anger, or even rage that we feel.

Being angry doesn't mean that your children are out-of-control or that they are not coping well. Anger is a legitimate response to the unfairness of life and should be acknowledged. If you as the parent can claim your right to feel cheated, it will be easier for your children to express these normal feelings. To try to suppress such feelings makes it harder to cope with daily living.

Do not assume that if your child is not acting angry, everything is fine. Children often try to protect their parents from how they are really feeling. We all do this to one degree or another with people we love. Parents can ask their children if they ever feel angry that this is happening to their family. Reassure your children that there are times when you also feel angry at the unfairness of life. Tell them that talking about it may make them feel better. What's often underneath the anger is a profound sadness which needs to be shared in order to go on with daily life. This can be very painful to express and hear. Getting those feelings out into the open can help to diminish the power of such strong emotions, and help people regroup and feel less isolated.

Depending on the age of your children, you might want to plan for ways to distract them from focusing on the possibility of death. You can ask for help from people in your family or support network. It may be easier for someone else to listen to the children's distress and to give them an emotional break from the worry that their parent may not survive. Neither parents nor children should constantly think that things won't go well. You will need to plan strategies to keep the family going and to find ways to enjoy each other in spite of the illness.

Helping Your Children Cope

Managing your children's reactions when you have so little energy is probably the toughest part about dealing with progressive disease and its impact on children. There may be days you don't seem to have an ounce of extra energy to spare. There may be days when it's hard enough to figure out how you are going to get through it yourself, let alone deal with what your children may be feeling. The ages of your children will influence how you respond to their needs. Younger children who need a great deal of attention may seem harder to manage than those who are more self-sufficient. All children, however, will have needs that you may feel little energy to fulfill.

Try not to feel guilty about having cancer or not being able to meet everyone's needs. No one wills it on him or herself, and guilt hinders your ability to cope. You can let people know you are distressed, but point out that it is not your fault that you are sick. If it were someone else in your family that was ill, would you be there for them? The answer is probably yes, as stressful as it may be to deal with relationships that are tested by serious illness. So, don't apologize for being sick. Let people know how tough this time is and ask for their help in getting through the rough times together.

Your family circumstances will be critical in figuring out how to get through a difficult time. The more supportive family members that are available, the easier it will be to fill in the sick parent's role functions. Even in such families, every family member will feel more pressure to keep things going. Everyone should take an honest look at how they are managing the extra responsibilities. If you are the patient, you may suspect that your spouse or children are feeling tired and even resentful at times. That is to be expected even though people find it hard to admit. The anger is probably not directed at you, rather it's about the situation. There will be times when everyone's patience is at a low ebb. It's best not to try pretending that everything is normal. Do whatever you can to recognize that people may be unusually stressed and that you acknowledge their stress.

It's a good idea to let your children be involved in your daily routines (see Chapter 2). Are there small jobs that your children might do for you that will make them feel as if they are included in a special way? Can they make you a cup of tea after school, bring your medicines to the bedroom for you, retrieve or sort the mail if you're not feeling up to it? Children enjoy having special jobs for which you can offer praise. Being able to help you helps them feel special in your eyes and to feel good about themselves.

Others Can Help

In families that have a large support network, this kind of situation is more manageable because there are more people to help. However, the number of people is not the only criteria. Some families are used to pitching in to help one another while others may not be as close. It may be very difficult to ask for help. In fact, this is often the hardest part of managing a chronic illness. People like to be self-sufficient and take care of their own problems. However, cancer will sorely test self-reliance. There will probably be times when it's essential for your family's well being that you ask for help.

Since your cancer has recurred, it may be difficult for you to ask for help. If that is the case, is there someone in your family that can organize things for you? That person might assume the role of "coordinator" for you.

- Make a list of the things that need to be accomplished. You and your family will certainly be less stressed if the burdens of advanced cancer can be shared with people who care about you.
- Identify someone who can easily pick your children up from an activity that their children also attend.
- Determine if there are other people who can be asked to help during an emergency if they are unable to assume a more permanent job.

- Access your resource network. Is there a stay-at-home mom who shops for her family every Thursday morning and can she call Wednesday evening to see if you are running short on something?
- When people say to you "let me know what I can do," answer the question concretely depending on what is going on. If you are vague about your needs because you're not comfortable asking for help, nothing is achieved.
- Speak up when someone offers help. People usually mean it when they offer to help. In fact, it gives them satisfaction to be able to do something for someone they care about.

The Impact of Cancer on Your Children's Future

Many parents worry that the experience of advanced cancer may leave their children emotionally damaged. The experience will certainly have an impact, but it should not be assumed that this will be permanently damaging to children. If you do your best to be honest with your children and maintain as much normalcy in their lives as possible, there's a good chance of helping them get through the experience. In certain cases, some may even gain some benefits.

There are many forces that influence how your children will grow and develop into adulthood. These are genetic, social class, culture, personality, education, spiritual orientation, and the quality of child/parent relationships. Even when they have all of those things going for them, there are some that are never able to really take full advantage of all of their resources. There are others who, in spite of the most chaotic environments, achieve way beyond what might be expected. So it's hard to generalize about how the experience of chronic illness will impact them for an entire lifetime.

Most parents do the very best they can to deal with a cancer diagnosis and treatment, and that is really all that should be realistically expected. Unfortunately, people are rarely satisfied with their best efforts. It is easy to feel guilty and worry about what the experience of cancer will do to their child's future. It may help to remember that children are very resilient. If you find yourself in turmoil about how you or your children are doing, it would probably make sense to consider getting some help (see Chapter 3). For many people, especially those young enough to have children still living at home, this is probably the most stressful or serious situation they have ever encountered. It is not reasonable to expect a young family to intuitively know how to deal with all of the problems associated with advanced cancer.

Hands-On Tools

Many of the hands-on tools we suggested for using with your children in Chapters 1, 2, and 5 are useful here as well. Not all of the exercises will be right for your children. Just as with activities in the other chapters, select the ones that are most appropriate for your children. You are the best judge of what may help, and you can adapt them any way you see fit. At this point, you may feel more compelled to be sure that your children will have good memories of you, so many of these exercises lend themselves well to this.

◆ ***Leave a lasting legacy*** by helping your children write, tell, or draw stories about your times together can be healing for all of you. An easy way to do this is to make a scrapbook, journal, or memory album. You might choose to focus on a special activity that you did with each child. Or, you may prefer to make a family tree book and tell about people in your family. If this seems too hard, let your children pick out pictures and make their own picture book of memories. If you are too exhausted, ask a friend, school counselor, or family member to help. You may want to get your children to work on special journals for kids whose parents are ill (see Resource Guide).

◆ ***Read stories together that focus on feelings,*** which can be very therapeutic for children. Young children enjoy, *I Am So Mad* by Mercer Mayer. Older children can read aloud from fantasy stories such as *The Never Ending Story* or *The Chronicles of Narnia*. Stories are great because they indirectly show ways of sharing feelings and coping.

◆ ***Tell joint stories,*** which is another activity that requires less energy. You might begin with "Remember when we..." and let the children fill in blanks. Each of you can share favorite activities. You can use a tape recorder so your children will have a permanent record.

◆ ***Show your children how to make a mobile*** by having them write words for feelings they are having right now on the different pieces of paper or cardboard. Then they can color the pieces and attach them to a wire clothes hanger with string or yarn. You can talk to them about how many mixed emotions there are at a time like this, and how they change and move at different times.

◆ ***Make a necklace or badge of courage*** with your children. If they use beads, the beads could represent worries or hopes. One five-year-old showed her mom the bracelet she had made and told her that the large beads were for her big worries about her mom's cancer. If they use construction paper, they can draw pictures on them (or tape pictures from magazines) of things that make them feel strong. You can suggest they wear what they made when they are feeling scared, lonely, or sad.

◆ ***Suggest your children make something special*** for the parent or support person who does not physically have cancer. It could be a hat with words and pictures on it, or a piece of jewelry.

◆ ***Give your children a picture of yourself*** to glue on a piece of poster board. Tell them they can create a banner, sign, or poster with slogans they think would help you feel better. They can draw pictures or use pictures from magazines to attach to the board.

CHAPTER SEVEN

Special Issues

We have discussed the impact of cancer on children, parents, and families in general, however, every family is different and has its own circumstances. There may be certain family situations that make a diagnosis of cancer more difficult to manage. Single parent and non-traditional families face unique pressures and challenges. There are also families that have special problems, such as those facing marital or financial instability, or substance abuse issues. This chapter highlights some ways to address family concerns in these and other particular circumstances.

Single Parent Households

When a parent in a two-parent family becomes ill, the other parent is usually available as back up in the home, but that is not the case for single parents. Single parent households can experience special challenges when the primary caretaker is diagnosed with cancer. The mechanics of managing day-to-day demands of the illness, such as getting to treatment, arranging childcare, and paying medical bills can be difficult. These pressures are added to the normal family responsibilities of preparing meals, car-pooling, shopping, and meeting all of the family's other emotional and physical needs. This can be overwhelming, especially if you are feeling frightened and sick.

Single parents often feel like they are both the mother and father to their children and a diagnosis of cancer can add stress to the system. If the family has gone through a divorce or is in the midst of that process, life can seem all the more stressful. Whatever the situation, the children have already gone through the loss of the parent who is not living in the household. This can sometimes cause children to worry more about the well being of the parent they are living with and who will care for them if something happens.

If you are in this situation, talking to your children about the arrangements is especially important. Let them know that they do not need to worry about who would take care of them. Tell them you will make those arrangements for their care even if you are very sick. Because you are the only parent in the household, your children need to be reassured that they will not be left alone and that there will be someone there for them. You should plan to make legal arrangements for custody or guardianship should the need arise.

Plan to arrange for one or two people who can take over some of the care-taking responsibilities. You may already know who you can call upon. If you do not have the kind of support system that would provide a natural solution to this issue, there are social service agencies that can help people identify possible caretakers (see Chapter 3). Make it clear to your children that these people are only helping out temporarily. If you have been divorced, but the other parent is entering into the picture, let your children know that this is also just a temporary situation (see pages 157–159).

Your children should also be well versed in how to handle emergency procedures, since resources may be spread thinner. Of course, every child should know these procedures. But, it is good to have a back up plan for situations that may require immediate attention. For example, a seven-year-old child was alone in the house when his father became very ill. Fortunately the child had been taught how to call 911, and the paramedics were able to reach his father in time.

Since there is no other adult in the household, the tendency to turn to children for emotional support is always a possibility. While a parent doesn't intend to do this, sometimes it happens without awareness. With a chronic illness like cancer, the danger of reversing roles with children is real. The single parent needs more help in maintaining the household, and has more needs for emotional support. Children can start assuming more responsibility than is appropriate for their age and stage of development. Single parents need to consider who in their network of friends and relatives can be called upon to be there for emotional and practical support. Usually, being aware of the possibility of relying more on children than is appropriate for their age is enough to guard against this.

If the noncustodial parent is the one who is ill, the child may feel less connected to that parent, and therefore unable to really participate in the illness experience. Efforts should still be made to have the child remain involved with the ill parent.

Parents Without Partners

Parents Without Partners is an international, nonprofit membership organization devoted to the welfare and interests of single parents and their children. Single parents include divorced, never married, separated, and widowed parents. There are approximately 400 chapters that run programs balanced among three areas:

- educational activities
- family activities
- adult social and recreational activities

Parents Without Partners, Inc.
1650 South Dixie Highway
Suite 500
Boca Raton, FL 33432

Toll-free: 800-637-7974

Web site: www.parentswithoutpartners.org

છલ

Issues for Non-Traditional Families

Much of what has already been discussed about the needs of children when a parent is ill with cancer can be applied to other family situations. For children living in a gay or lesbian household, the issues can sometimes be more complex. Legal custody or guardianship may become an issue if the custodial parent is hospitalized or unavailable. A guardian, either temporary or permanent, needs to be designated to act on the child's behalf in the event of a parent's absence or in an emergency.

In a gay or lesbian household, children may already feel they are different from their peers. They may have felt the effects of prejudice or homophobia. Adding a cancer diagnosis to this situation can result in children feeling very different from their peers. It can also be more complicated if extended families are not supportive or have no contact with the couple.

Parents who are homosexual have probably already explained this to their children. So, the same advice they give to their children about being different can also apply to the new situation of having a parent with cancer. Talking with children about these circumstances in a matter-of-fact way is the best approach. Children often handle this better than adults, and better than anticipated. If the homosexuality has been kept a secret or has not been openly discussed with the children, however, there may be additional tension when an illness enters the picture. While the parents may have been able to maintain their confidentiality and privacy within the community, this is more difficult when medical illness occurs.

For children in gay or lesbian families, the emotional issues may also be influenced by whether divorce is a part of their history, a single parent has adopted them, or the parent has undergone artificial insemination. If they have experienced the break-up of a two-parent household, their feelings of grief about the divorce may recur and be more intense. The crisis of a cancer diagnosis can bring up old feelings of loss as the child's world is suddenly threatened by the illness of the custodial parent. Custodial parents may want to pay special attention if their children seem more insecure during this time. If the noncustodial parent maintains a close relationship, extra visits might be helpful to reassure children that they still have two parents who love them. Sometimes, unresolved parental anger and feelings of betrayal may have complicated the divorce. In this case, keeping these feelings outside of the relationship with the children is a healthy approach. Otherwise, this will make it harder for the whole family to get through the crisis of a cancer diagnosis.

Adopted children often face questions about self-worth as they mature and try to figure out who they are in relation to the parents they have not grown up with. A diagnosis of cancer could result in adopted children feeling more insecure than usual and they may need special reassurance that they will be cared for if anything should happen to their adoptive parent.

The quality and availability of a support network can make a difference in the ability of non-traditional families to cope with this experience. If a supportive network does not exist, talk to the hospital social worker about other resources. In many gay communities, special support programs exist, with therapists who are familiar with the special needs of this population. If a parent is not already familiar with these resources, look into what is available in the event that counseling is needed to help feel as secure as possible during this period of family upheaval.

When the Household Has Special Problems

Marital Instability

A diagnosis of cancer can challenge all marriages, even those that may have seemed solid, but especially marriages that are troubled. The struggle with a life-threatening disease can boil a marriage down to its essence, and show you and your spouse what issues are affecting your relationship. Indeed, some couples must reach a state of relationship crisis before they can confront the issues that are affecting the marriage, and cancer can help to bring about just such a crisis. The question is what effect this turbulence will ultimately have on the marriage.

For some couples, a bout with a serious illness such as cancer can actually strengthen and enhance relationships, and may help a shaky marriage steady its course. A life-threatening situation can put more trivial conflicts into perspective and lead to a reevaluation of life's priorities. You may find that your family, including your spouse, "closes ranks" around you to support you during your diagnosis and recovery. All these elements of fighting a serious illness may provide an opportunity for reconciliation. However, you should not look for a "fairy tale" change in a troubled relationship. If a marriage is to be healed at any time, it will likely be the result of hard work. Success will depend on open communication and brave confrontation of painful issues. You may even find marital counseling or other professional help to be necessary as you and your spouse work to heal the relationship (see Chapter 3).

Unfortunately, the stress of dealing with cancer can also push a troubled marriage to the breaking point. In general, the rate of separation or divorce is no different when someone has cancer than at any other time. But, the stress of treatment and recovery can certainly precipitate the inevitable. This is especially true in relationships where partners have poor communication and coping skills.

It may come to pass, then, that you and your spouse realize that separation or divorce is inevitable. The question then becomes when you should separate. The timing of the split is complicated by the cancer diagnosis and recovery and what effects the separation will have on the children. It is preferable to plan the separation to occur at the best time for the children. The appropriate timing for your family will of course depend on your individual circumstances. If the situation is explosive, then immediate separation may be best. This is especially true if there is verbal or physical abuse in the household, or if the strain is causing difficulties in recovery for the person with cancer.

In families where the tension is under control and the couple is able to maintain a civil relationship, it may benefit the children to postpone a separation until other upheavals in the family are handled. In most cases, the best choice for the children may be for the couple to get through the illness before separating. In this way, top priority can be given to the children and to the ill parent's recovery before introducing yet more upheaval into the family. The children are spared having to deal with multiple traumas at the same time. Then, the ill parent is able to focus on his or her recovery without the additional stress of divorce proceedings.

When the children must be told about the impending separation or divorce, it is very important to make clear that the two events of cancer and the marital problems are completely separate and unrelated events, and that one did not cause the other. Explain to your children that your marriage had problems before cancer even came into the picture. They may otherwise come to the conclusion that illnesses can cause people to leave, or that problems in relationships can lead to illness. They may also blame themselves for the breakup of the relationship. It may help to take advantage of professional counseling now to help your children cope with the multiple stresses that they are experiencing (see Chapter 3).

If separation had already occurred, or if one parent had already started to withdraw from the household when the cancer diagnosis or treatment occurred, it may become necessary for that spouse to become more involved in the household again, and to help pick up some of the parental tasks. For children, this change can be both confusing and difficult. It is very important to make it clear to the children that this does not indicate that the marriage has been revived or that the estranged parent is coming back permanently. Explain to the children that this situation is temporary, so they don't begin to hold false hopes. Otherwise, they may experience just as much trauma the second time the estranged spouse withdraws from the household as they did the first time.

Financial Instability

The costs related to cancer treatment can be substantial, especially for a family who lives on a limited budget. In addition to the high costs of hospitalization and treatment, there are hidden costs that can come from travel to and from treatment, housekeeping costs, and increased childcare needs. The person with cancer may have to take considerable time off from work. There also may be understandable temptations to spend money on things that will ease you and your family through the cancer experience. You may find that you are having financial difficulties, which adds to your stress.

It would not be unusual for an already stressed family to choose to be in denial about their financial situation, or at least postpone dealing with the situation until after recovery from cancer. However, if you find yourself in such a situation, it is crucial that you take a deep breath and face your financial crisis head on. Financial problems have a way of growing even more out of control if neglected. In addition, there are resources that should be taken advantage of as soon as possible because they may only be available to you during or just after your illness. Your cancer center may have a special fund to help patients in severe need or your social worker may be able to appeal to private foundations or donors to help. Your local community or church may do a fund raising drive to help you through this time.

Don't be afraid to ask for help. You may pride yourself on never having had to fall back on financial assistance before, but cancer has made your situation exceptional, and there are programs and services available especially to help families like yours through these hard times. Remember that your situation is temporary, and one that others have weathered. In the future, you may be the one in a position to offer financial help to someone else in difficulty.

Keep in mind that your children may be more aware of the family financial problems than you might think. They may overhear, for example, arguments that you might have with your spouse about money. Children do not need the extra burden of worrying about money when they have already been worrying about a sick parent. Your children need to be reassured that your family is not in such dire straits that you will not have enough to eat or a place to live. Besides taking action to get your finances in control, take time to assure your children that you're all going to be okay, while keeping conversations about money worries in the household minimal. If it becomes necessary to explain financial limitations to your children, keep it light and practical, with an emphasis on the temporary nature of your circumstances.

Money Matters

A good resource to consider when getting your finances in order is the *Taking Charge of Money Matters* workshop and pamphlet offered by the American Cancer Society's I CAN COPE program. This series offers financial guidance for cancer survivors and their families. Topics include the fundamentals of insurance, estate planning, returning to work, disability insurance, how to improve your financial planning, financial resources, and how to create a budget. Call 800-ACS-2345 to learn more about this program.

෯෯

Sources of Financial Help

You have several options for getting assistance with financial problems. Possible sources of help and relief for families in financial need include:

- Income assistance for low-income families through Supplemental Security Insurance (SSI) benefits
- Income assistance for non-working parents from the Aid to Families with Dependent Children (AFDC) program
- Help with travel, meals, and lodging from public and private programs
- Assistance with basic living costs (rent, mortgage, insurance premiums, utilities, telephone) from public and private programs
- Help from church, civic, social, and fraternal groups in the community
- General help from special funds in the medical center or community
- Assistance from targeted fundraising for an individual patient or family
- Low-interest loans from family or friends
- Drug assistance programs
- Home equity conversion
- Declaration of bankruptcy

Your hospital social worker or a financial assistance planner can be helpful in guiding you through the often complicated process of accessing financial resources.

৩৫

Alcoholism or Drug Abuse in the Home

Families that were already dealing with alcoholism or substance abuse in the home may have been chaotic, unpredictable, and significantly distressed before cancer even came into the picture. The presence of a serious disease can complicate what is already a difficult situation. However, in some cases, the presence of a life-threatening disease can serve as a "wake-up call" and lead to a temporary improvement. In other cases, the substance abuse problem may be made worse by the cancer diagnosis. People may use substances more in this case in an attempt to avoid the reality of the situation.

What Are the Signs of a Problem?

How can you tell whether you, or someone close to you, may have a drinking problem? Answering the following four questions can help you find out. (To help remember these questions, note that the first letter of a key word in each of the four questions spells "CAGE.")

- Have you ever felt you should **C**ut down on your drinking?
- Have people **A**nnoyed you by criticizing your drinking?
- Have you ever felt bad or **G**uilty about your drinking?
- Have you ever had a drink first thing in the morning to steady your nerves or to get rid of a hangover (**E**ye opener)?

One "yes" response suggests a possible alcohol problem. If you or a family member responded "yes" to more than one question, it is highly likely that a problem exists. In either case, it is important that you get follow-up for yourself or the family member as soon as possible. A doctor or other health care provider can make a recommendation about the best course of action.

Even if you answered "no" to all of the above questions, if you are encountering drinking-related problems with your job, relationships, health, or with the law, you should still seek professional help. The effects of alcohol abuse can be extremely serious—even fatal—both to you and to others.

Source: Alcoholism: Getting the Facts. NIH Publication No. 96-4153. Rockville, MD., 1996.

୧ଓ

There are several risks to be aware of now if anyone in your family is fighting a substance abuse problem. If the parent who has cancer continues to engage in drinking or drug use, it will inhibit treatment and healing and compromise his or her health. If the well parent is the one who abuses drugs or alcohol, he or she may not be responsible for family obligations, and may even neglect the children. Physical hazards can be created by adults who are under the influence, both within the home and outside the home, especially while driving. There may be legal entanglements associated with substance abuse that can cause added stress to a family already under significant strain.

Another danger to be aware of is that adolescents in alcoholic homes tend to be at increased risk of initiating substance use. The crisis of cancer in the home may make them even more likely to start using alcohol or drugs as a way of escaping from the family's problems. If you think your teenager has started to use drugs or alcohol, consider having him or her speak with a trusted adult friend. If you don't feel up to such a talk right now, your teenager might be more likely to confide in someone other than his or her parents. If the situation appears serious, consider getting professional help (see Chapter 3).

There are other steps you can take now to reduce the risks to your family that can be caused by substance abuse during cancer treatment and recovery. The highest priority should be protecting the health and emotional well being of the children in the household. Safety should always be put first, both within the home and during driving. If your spouse is abusing drugs, you may have to make alternative arrangements for childcare during your treatment. Consider having your children stay with your parents or other trusted relatives or friends. Even if you are normally able to compensate for your spouse's behaviors and protect the children, you may not currently have the inner resources needed to do so now. The added burden may also compromise your own recovery.

If children must stay in the home, you need to take steps to decrease the impact of your spouse's drinking or drug abuse. Avoid justifying your spouse's addictive behavior by blaming it on the cancer. Do not join your spouse in drinking or drug use—this will only compound your problems! Try instead to help your spouse focus on things that will help you, as a couple, manage the illness. Tell your spouse that you will be more able to deal with your cancer if he or she can control the alcohol or drug abuse. Urge your spouse to help get on the road to recovery. There are many support programs available, such as Alcoholics Anonymous, Al-Anon, or Alateen. The crisis of cancer may actually provide emotional energy for dealing with this problem.

Advice for the Well Spouse:
How You Can Cope Now

As you've probably discovered by now, as the well spouse, you'll have many responsibilities to assume. You'll find yourself taking care of your ill spouse, both physically and emotionally, acting as cheerleader, and advocate. In addition, you will be taking over many of the parenting duties and you will probably be serving as family spokesperson to the outside world. There will be many new changes and new routines. This will be in addition to all of the obligations that you had before.

A major change like this can be very disruptive. You will be dealing with a very complicated set of emotions. You will likely be feeling a great deal of sympathy for what your spouse is going through now and you will be worried about what the future will bring. You may be dwelling on the possibility of losing your spouse, and dealing with fears of abandonment. Anger at the unfairness of what has happened to you and your family may flair up from time to time. And even when you get some help and relief from family and friends, it may be difficult for you to feel like you can let go and relax for a little bit. It can be hard to let go of the guilt of getting away from the house when your spouse is sick at home. And of course, even when you do get away from the home, the cold reality of the situation can hit you the moment you come back through the door.

The first thing to keep in mind as you work to adapt to and cope with this situation is that you are a true hero! Be sure to give yourself ample credit for all that you are doing now. Think of how much it means to your family that you're giving it your best shot. That doesn't mean that you have to do everything perfectly. Pace yourself. Be sure to forgive yourself if you have to fall back on a little extra help at times. Let some things go and lower your standards. Try to be realistic about what you can and cannot accomplish by yourself. Find out who is available to help, and take advantage of their offers of assistance. It will help ease your burden greatly if you let people help. Delegate chores and errands to those people who want to help.

While the clear priority now is helping your spouse get through the cancer, it is very important that you take care of your own needs too. Taking care of yourself will ultimately benefit everyone. You are needed to maintain an even keel during these tough times. When you get help from friends and family, be sure to use that time to take a respite for yourself. Take time away from the household to do something that replenishes you. This can be tough at times because your spouse may be envious of your health and ability to be active. But, try not to let that stop you from taking the time you need.

It may also help to seek emotional support from people that are outside of the household. It can be soothing to find someone you can confide in, someone who can listen and support you emotionally, and who can understand the anger and resentment you may be feeling now. Suppressing such emotions can be exhausting. The benefit is that you gain energy when you release some of your frustration, sadness, and anger. You might even consider joining a support group for caregivers, where you'll find others who can truly relate to what you're going through now (see the Well Spouse Foundation in the Resource Guide). They may be able to offer helpful advice on how you and your family can get through these tough times with some degree of comfort and sense of well being.

A Caregiver's Advice

"As a caregiver, your life is not going to be the same. It is essential that you maintain a healthy, high-quality level of physical and mental fitness so that you can still carry on with your life, while also helping the one in treatment. Find compassionate and understanding friends with whom you can talk to relieve your stress. In short, take care of yourself at the same time, paying attention to diet, exercise, and sleep requirements, to better help others and yourself. While being realistic, try to remain optimistic."

When Children Are Facing Other Losses

Life can deal some hard blows, and children are not exempt from painful realities. While your family is dealing with cancer, your children also may have other major life stresses. They may have even lost a close family member, such as a grandparent that succumbs to old age. For a child, especially one who is already aware of the seriousness of the parent's cancer, such an event can really bring home the reality and finality of death.

There are several issues to keep in mind if you are now helping your children cope with the death of someone close to them. You can expect your children's reactions to this loss to be magnified by the presence of cancer in the household. For example, your children may perceive that lightning has "struck twice." They may feel that illness and death have targeted their world, which may lead to insecurity. Your children may also become more afraid of the cancer, and more fearful of what the outcome will be.

It is crucial that you take the time now to talk with your children about this loss, to help them work through grief. The advice you read about in Chapter 6 will guide you in helping your child adapt to this loss. Help your children see these concurrent misfortunes as independent events. Make it clear to them that there is no relationship between the recent death that has occurred and the parent's illness. It's important that your children are able to differentiate between these two events. If you haven't already had to explain about the unfairness of life that we all eventually discover, now may be a good time. If you feel, however, that your children are still having a very difficult time adapting to these circumstances, do not hesitate to get help (see Chapter 3).

AIDS-Related Cancers

If your cancer is AIDS-related, you may encounter misunderstanding and prejudice. You may find that you become isolated from your family and friends. Sadly, AIDS still carries a stigma in most communities. This stigma can cloud the whole family if the presence of AIDS in your household becomes known. Your children may be kept from playing with friends and be ostracized at school and other social settings. Older children, especially, may even have a fearful response to the presence of AIDS in their home. This leaves you with a difficult question: Should you tell your children that you or your spouse has AIDS? Or would it be better to tell them about the cancer and other specific illnesses that may arise without explaining that AIDS is the cause?

There is no one correct answer to this question—you will have to make a decision based on your family's individual circumstances. But, there are several factors that can help you to decide how much to tell your children. One of the most important considerations is the age of the children. For toddlers and young schoolchildren, there is probably no harm in not using the word AIDS. If you do use this term, and they are too young to understand its implications, they may innocently repeat it in less than ideal circumstances. It may be best, with younger children, to explain AIDS-related illnesses in very simple terms such as, "Daddy has a very serious skin problem" or "Mommy has something wrong with her blood." Older children, on the other hand, have usually been exposed to at least some information about HIV and AIDS, and can understand the syndrome better. Indeed, they may put two and two together and wonder if it's AIDS when they learn of the specific symptoms of the ill parent. With older children and teenagers, then, it's usually appropriate to be straightforward with them about the AIDS diagnosis.

Also consider that if several other family members (or even people outside of the family) know about the diagnosis, the children might well hear about it from someone other than you. They may feel betrayed if they feel that their parents have been less than honest with them. Under such circumstances, it is probably best to be candid with the children, before they hear it from another source. Honesty is also the best policy if your children ask you directly if you or your spouse has AIDS. If they are sophisticated enough to even ask, chances are they already have a pretty good idea of what's going on.

If you have told your children about the AIDS, you will also need to tell them this is private family information. Tell them this should not be shared with anybody outside the household. You'll have to tell your children that others are often more afraid of the disease than they should be. Because they do not understand it, they might not treat your children well if they find out. Tell your children who they can talk to about the AIDS in your family, so they have someone to go to when they are upset.

You should also take this opportunity to give your children more information about the disease itself, to keep them from having their own misconceptions. Explain to your children that AIDS is not easy to catch and they have nothing to fear from touching or kissing Mommy (or Daddy). You'll have to explain to them, in age-appropriate terms, how HIV/AIDS is transmitted, so it does not remain a scary mystery to them. You'll also probably field some tough questions from your children now—the toughest one probably being, "Doesn't everyone die from AIDS?" You'll have to explain to your children that it's true that there is no real cure for AIDS now, but assure them that scientists are working very hard to find a cure. In the meantime, the good news is that there are now very good treatments available that can help people with AIDS live for a long time.

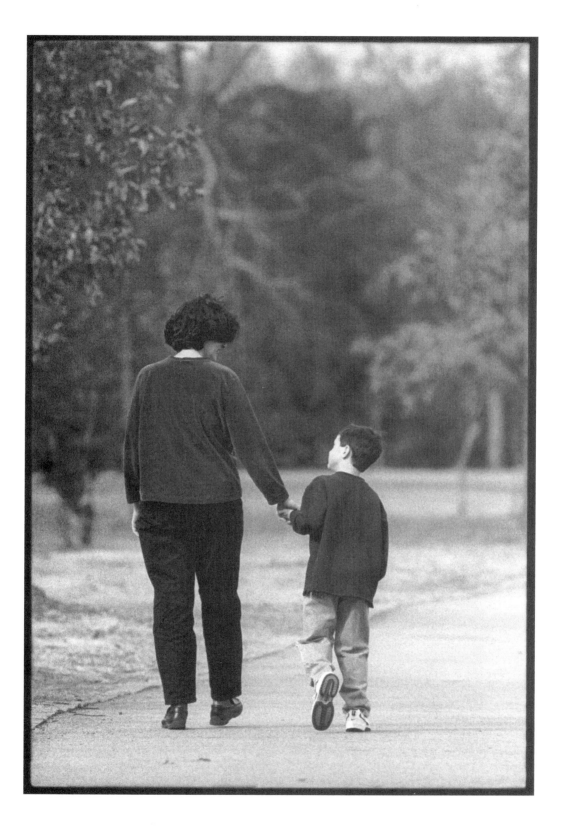

Kids' Corner

How to Use This Workbook

If your Mom or Dad has been diagnosed with cancer, it affects you and everyone else in your family. There are lots of changes happening that might make you worry or become upset. It can be hard when your parent is sick. Sometimes kids and teens can be confused by many different thoughts and feelings. This workbook can help you understand and talk about what it is like to have a parent with cancer.

Most kids, teens, and parents will view this workbook as private. You should ask your parents to respect your privacy. This means they will only look at it if you tell them to. But, you may find that sharing parts of it will make it easier for you to bring your thoughts and feelings out into the open. Then you can listen to what they have on their minds too. It's good to share these things at times like this. You also may want to use this workbook to talk with a teacher, counselor, or other trusted adult.

You can use this workbook to keep track of things after you first learned about your Mom or Dad's diagnosis, through treatment, and the time following treatment.

You
can use this workbook
no matter how old you are.

If you are a teenager, at first glance you may think this workbook will not be useful to you. However, let your playful self have fun with the exercises. Being creative is a great way to relieve stress. If you have younger brothers and sisters, you might also help them with the activities. Sharing can make you closer. Also, doing the activities will help you understand yourself in ways that may surprise you.

If you have questions or worries
ABOUT ANYTHING,
please
talk to your Mom and Dad.

It helps to let them know how you feel. That can help you feel better too. Understanding each other's feelings can make you all feel closer.

The feeling Clock

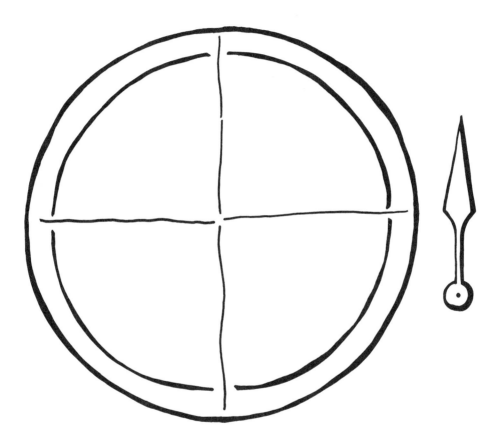

Directions: Just as a real clock tells time, this clock tells feelings. Like a real clock that changes time, this clock changes feelings. Think about feelings as mad, sad, glad, or scared. We can usually put our feelings into one of these categories. Use crayons or markers to color each of the four areas on the clock. We suggest you use red for mad, blue for sad, yellow for glad, and green for scared. Cut out the circle and the hand for the clock. Attach the hand (arrow) to the clock with a small metal fastener. Now point the arrow to the feeling that you are having right now about your Mom or Dad's cancer. You can use the clock to let people know how you are feeling. You can even move the clock's hands to the feelings you would like to have in the future.

You might want to ask your brothers, sisters, or parents to make a clock and put their name on it. You can mount the clocks on a family bulletin board or even the refrigerator.

T-Shirt Message

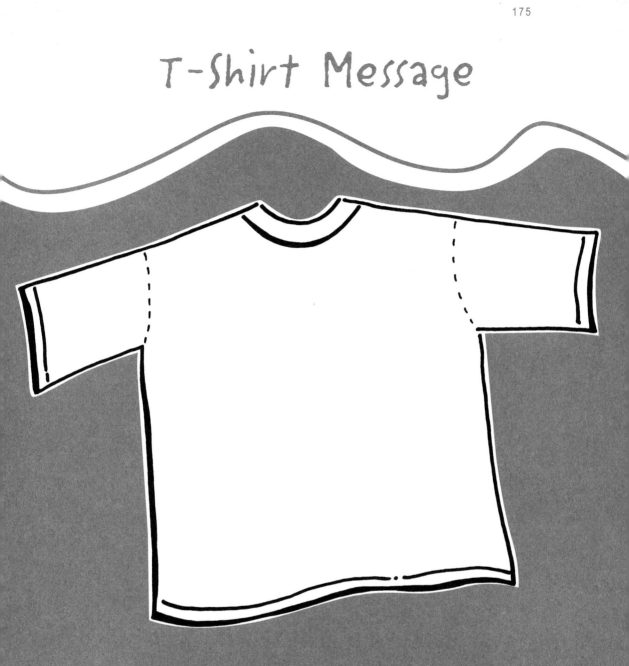

Directions: Think about how people put messages on bumper stickers and T-shirts. Use this outline to write your own message about what you think or feel about your parent having cancer.

Shield Slogans

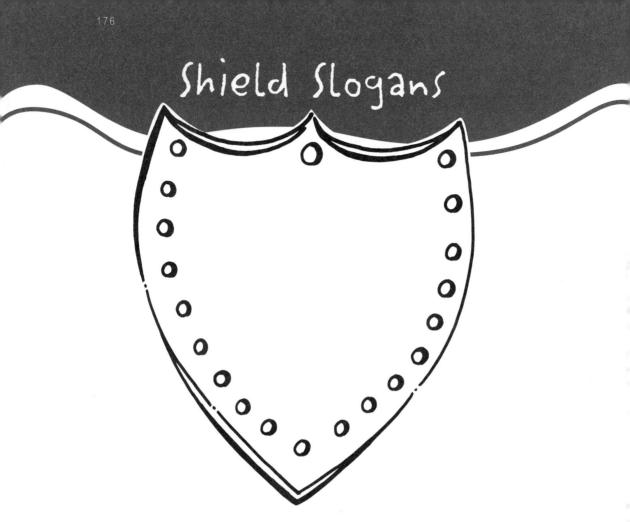

Directions: Make a shield out of cardboard and decorate. The out-side of the shield is for what you want to keep away from you. Write a slogan or phrase you can use for protection. You could write, "KEEP OUT." On the inside of the shield you can put what you want to keep close to you. You can write the names of people who support you or favorite activities.

Computer Screen-Saver Message

Directions: Many people put special messages or thoughts on their computer screens. If you could make a screen saver thought about your parent's cancer, what would it be? Try to write a message about your biggest concern. If you have a computer in the family, you might put the message on the screen saver for a few days, or ask your parents to do that for you.

Journal or Scrapbook

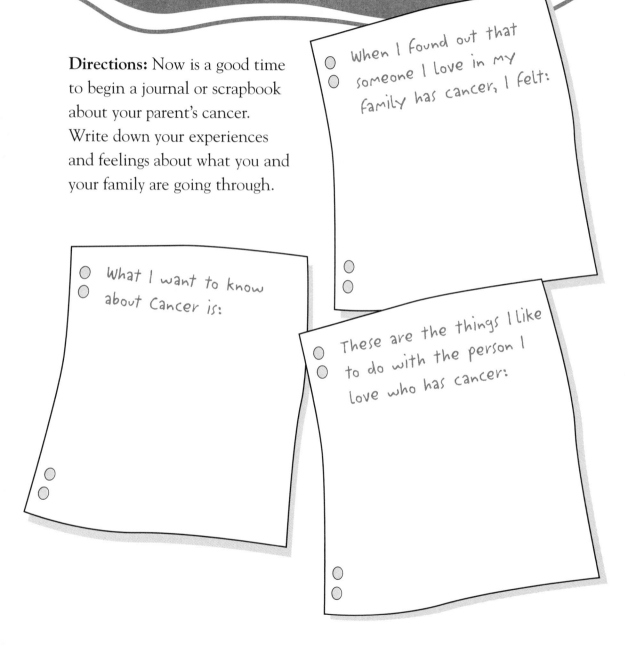

Directions: Now is a good time to begin a journal or scrapbook about your parent's cancer. Write down your experiences and feelings about what you and your family are going through.

When I found out that someone I love in my family has cancer, I felt:

What I want to know about Cancer is:

These are the things I like to do with the person I love who has cancer:

Kids Can Help

Directions: Color a square each time you help out with one of the jobs below.

Wash Dishes						
Fold Clothes						
Put Toys Away						
Make Bed						
Take Out Garbage						
Feed Pet						

feeling Pictures

This is how I look when I am:

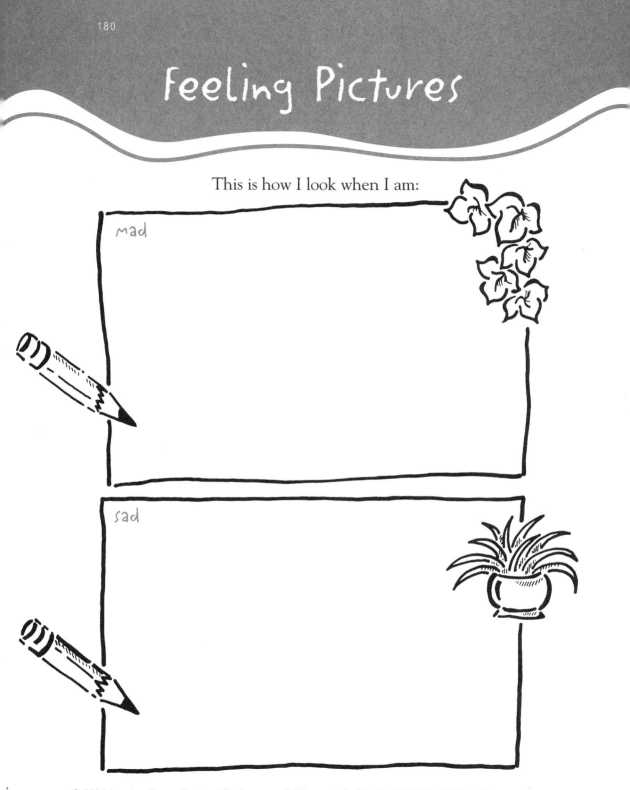

mad

sad

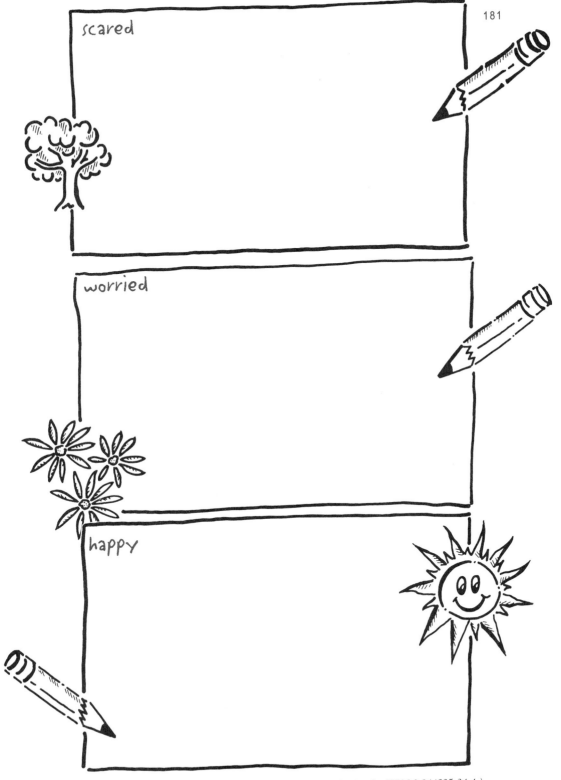

scared

worried

happy

Story Time

Directions: Write a story or poem for the person you love who is in the hospital or getting treatment.

About Treatment

Directions: Draw a picture of your favorite doctor or nurse, or what the clinic, hospital or chemotherapy department looks like:

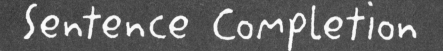

Sentence Completion

Directions: Draw or fill in the blanks.

What makes me feel good about my parent's cancer is:

What makes me feel bad about my parent's cancer is:

What I like most about my family is:

What I don't like about my parent being sick is:

Changes in the House

Directions: There have probably been many changes in your house since your parent became sick. People and things are always changing. Some rooms in your house may feel different. Mark the rooms that are different and explain what has changed.

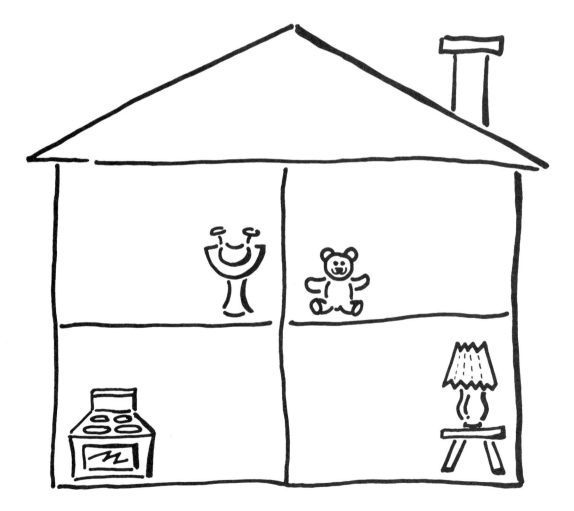

Family Tree

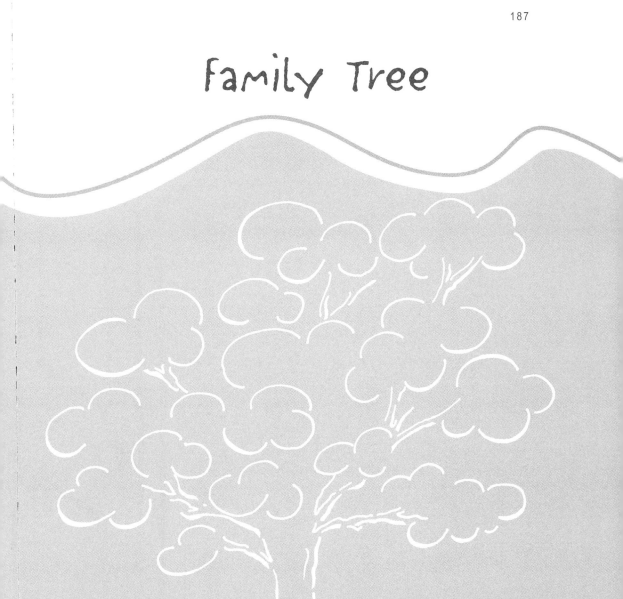

Directions: Decorate this tree with the things that make your family special. You might also ask your Mom or Dad to buy a small potted tree for your family to use to hang symbols of hope. Or, you can use branches you find on the ground outside and put them in a can with dirt and small rocks to hold the branches in place. You can hang notes with messages written on them, ribbons, hearts, or other special tokens and reminders of hope.

Door Design

Directions: Draw a picture to the left side of the door that shows what it was like before cancer, and a picture on the right side of the door to show what it is like after cancer.

BEFORE CANCER (Draw picture below)

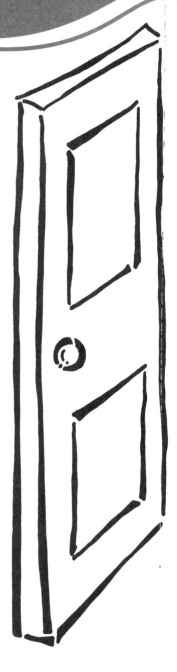

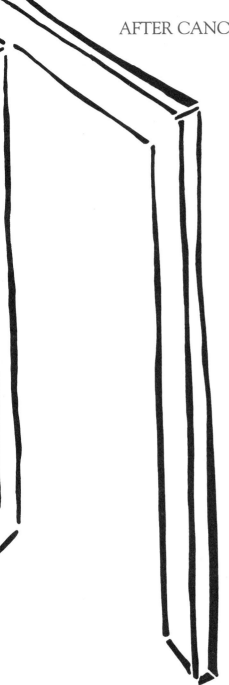

AFTER CANCER (Draw picture below)

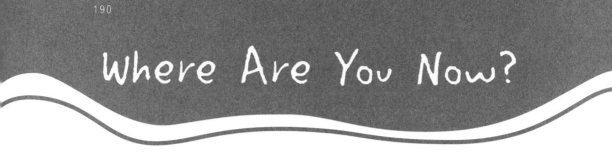

Where Are You Now?

Directions: When your parent or family member has finished treatment, write or draw answers to the following questions.

What was the easiest thing?

What was the hardest thing?

What were you most surprised about?

What do you want to know now?

What are you still worried about?

When Mommy or Daddy goes for a checkup, I feel:

Now that treatment is finished, this is how I feel:

Word Find

Directions: Circle the following words in the puzzle.

cell	treatment	symptom
nurse	medicine	hospital
chronic	doctor	tumor
body		

t	m	e	d	i	c	i	n	e	b
r	a	h	o	s	p	i	t	a	l
e	s	j	c	k	z	u	g	l	d
a	u	z	t	q	s	o	e	c	n
t	v	b	o	d	y	c	j	h	u
m	h	c	r	b	m	l	k	r	r
e	k	p	s	n	p	a	w	o	s
n	l	x	r	c	t	s	i	n	e
t	t	w	t	a	o	r	n	i	j
m	r	f	t	u	m	o	r	c	s

To-Do List

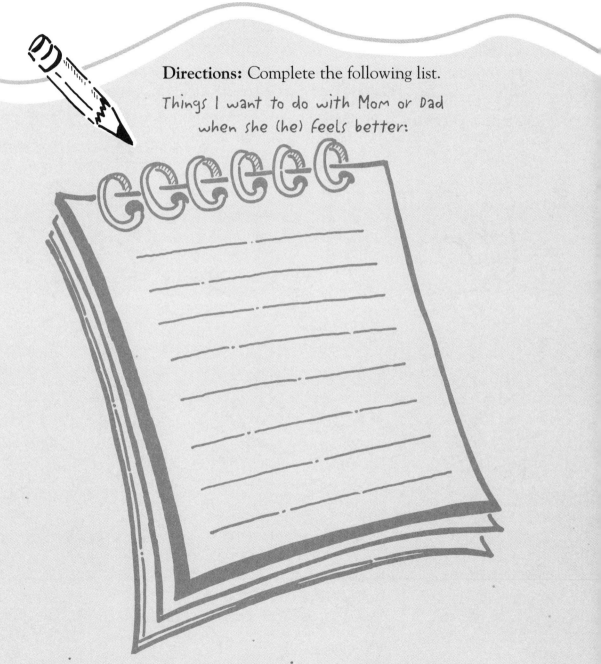

Directions: Complete the following list.

Things I want to do with Mom or Dad when she (he) feels better:

Keep Healthy

Directions: One way to stay healthy is to eat foods that are nutritious. Color in the foods below. Circle the foods that you like to eat, and star the ones that are really good for you.

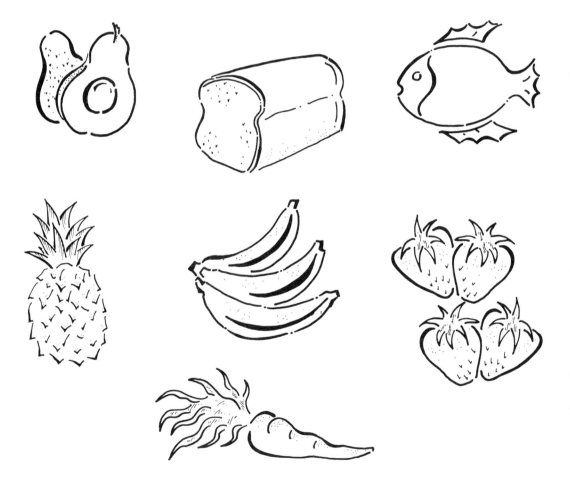

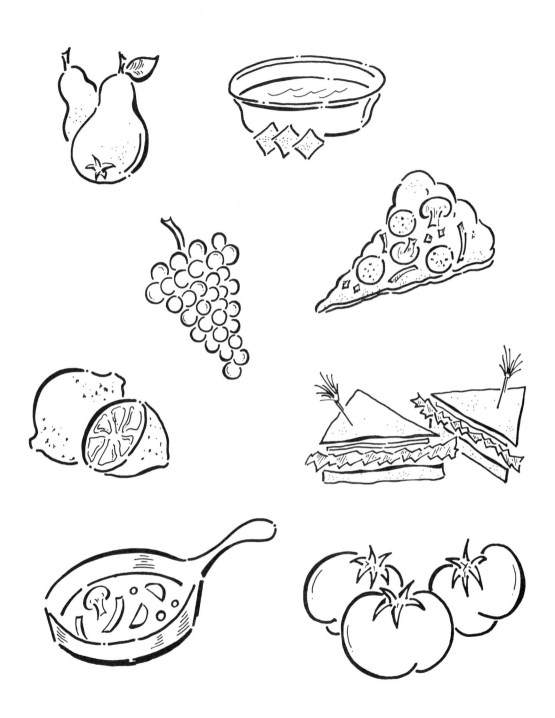

Word Scramble

Directions: Unscramble the letters to make words.

agcehn _____

mrout _____

ncarec _____

ahhyelt _____

ppyha _____

ovle _____

ctrodo _____

ifmlya _____

Answers:

1) change 2) tumor 3) cancer 4) healthy 5) happy 6) love 7) doctor 8) family

Building Blocks of Helpers

Directions: Draw a picture of the person who helps you with the things listed in each of the squares.

Someone I can talk to about my sick parent.

Someone who can answer my questions.

Someone who can fix something for me, like my bike.

Someone I can talk to about my feelings.

Someone I can have fun with.

Someone who can help me with my clothes, hair, etc.

Connect the Dots

Directions: Connect the dots to draw a picture that symbolizes hope.

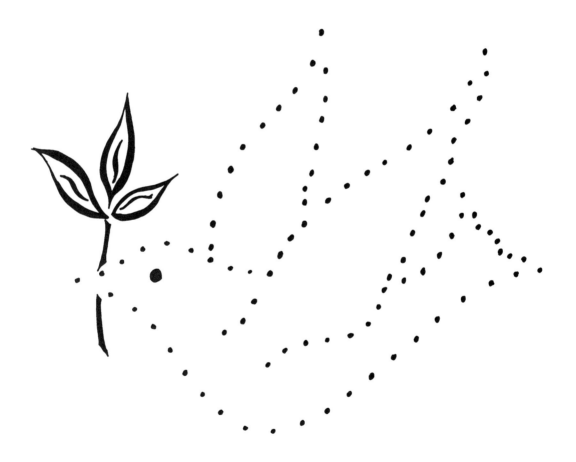

Find Healing

Directions: Fill in the blanks to find the path to healing.

Clues

H _ _ _ _ _ _ _   (Place where doctors & nurses work)

E _ _ _   (Test; physical)

A _ _ _ _ _   (Another word for scared)

L _ _ _ _   (These are used to breathe)

I _ _   (Another word for sick)

N _ _ _ _   (Person who works with doctors and is trained and licensed to care for people who are sick)

G _ _ _   (Something small that causes sickness or disease)

Answers:

1) Hospital 2) Exam 3) Afraid 4) Lungs 5) Ill 6) Nurse 7) Germ

Sentence Completion

Directions: Draw or fill in the blanks.

Since the cancer has come back, this is how I feel:

What I worry about most is:

What I look forward to is:

Picture of the future

Directions: Draw a picture of yourself and your family five years from now.

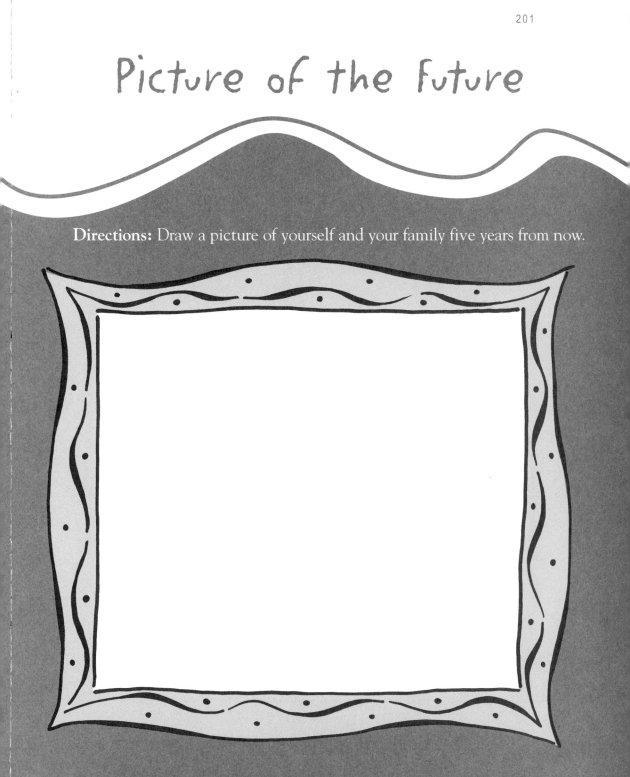

Wishes

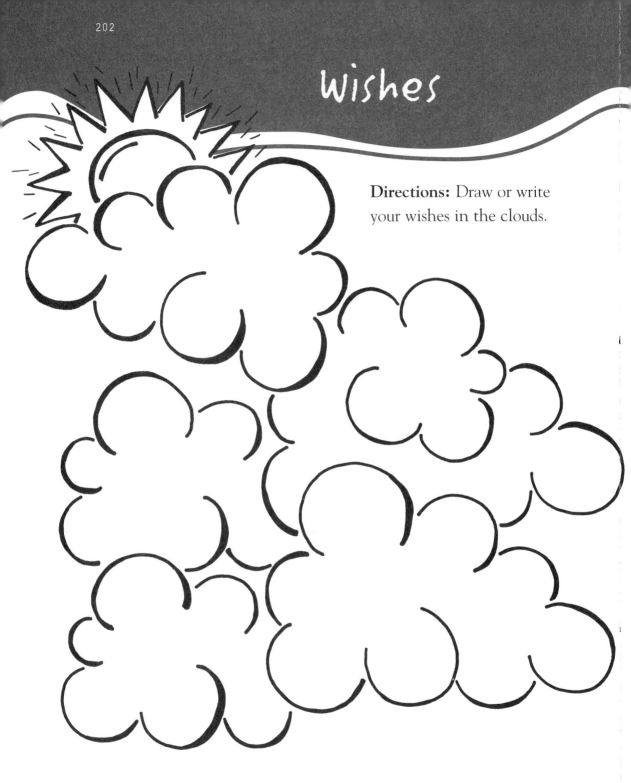

Directions: Draw or write your wishes in the clouds.

Resource Guide

Family Support and Services

**AMC Cancer Research Center
& Foundation**
1600 Pierce Street
Denver, CO 80214
Toll-free (Counseling): 800-525-3777
Phone: 303-239-3422
Fax: 303-233-1863
Web site: *http://www.amc.org*

Description: Through the counseling line
of this nonprofit research center, people
can request free publications and receive
answers to questions about cancer. The
web site contains an area about on-going
research and general information about
specific types of cancer.

Cancer Care, Inc.
275 Seventh Avenue
New York, NY 10001
Toll-free (Counseling): 800-813-HOPE
Phone: 212-302-2400
Fax: 212-719-0263
Web site: *http://www.cancercare.org*
Web site: *http://www.cancercare.org/
spanishmenu.htm* (Spanish version)

Description: A nonprofit social service
agency, Cancer Care, Inc. provides counseling and guidance to help people with cancer, their families, and friends cope with the
impact of cancer. The web site includes

detailed information on specific cancers and
cancer treatment, clinical trials, and links to
other sites. The organization also provides
videos, support groups (online, telephone,
and face-to-face), workshops, seminars and
clinics, a newsletter, and other publications
to interested consumers. *Spanish speaking
staff is also available.*

Centering Corporation
1531 North Saddle Creek Road
Omaha, NE 68104
Phone: 402-553-1200
Fax: 402-553-0507
Web site: *http://www.centering.org*

Description: The Centering Corporation
is a nonprofit bereavement resource center.
It provides books as well as audio and video
materials for all age groups on a wide range
of bereavement topics. Call to obtain a
free catalog listing of over 300 resources.

The Compassionate Friends
National Headquarters
P.O. Box 3696
Oakbrook, IL 60522-3696
Toll-free: 877-969-0010
Phone: 630-990-0010
Fax: 630-990-0246
Web site: *http://www.compassionate
friends.org*

Description: Compassionate Friends is a nationwide self-help organization offering support to families who have experienced the death of a child, of any age, from any cause. It publishes a newsletter and other materials on parent and sibling bereavement. It makes referrals to nearly 600 local chapters.

The Dougy Center, The National Center for Grieving Children and Families
P.O. Box 86852
Portland, OR 97286
Phone: 503-775-5683
Fax: 503-777-3097
Web site: *http://www.dougy.org*

Description: The Dougy Center is a nonprofit support center in Portland that was founded in 1982 to help grieving children, teens, and families. They also offer support and training locally, nationally, and internationally to individuals and organizations seeking to assist children and teens in grief.

Family Caregiver Alliance
690 Market Street, Suite 600
San Francisco, CA 94104
Phone: 415-434-3388
Fax: 415-434-3508
Web site: *http://www.caregiver.org*

Description: The Family Caregiver Alliance provides information and resources on long-term care. They also offer fact sheets, statistics, public policy statements, an online support group, and other links.

Gilda's Club
195 West Houston Street
New York, NY 10014
Toll-free: 888-445-3248
Phone: 212-647-9700
Web site: *http://gildasclub.org*

Description: Gilda's Club is a nonprofit organization providing a place where people with cancer and their families and friends join with others to build social and emotional support as a supplement to medical care. Services are free of charge and include support and networking groups, lectures and workshops, and social events.

They offer a program called, "Noogieland" for children with cancer and children whose parents have cancer.

Kids Konnected
27071 Cabot Road, Suite 102
Laguna Hills, CA 92653
Toll-free: 800-899-2866
Fax: 949-582-3983
Web site: *http://www.kidskonnected.org*

Description: Kids Konnected is a national, nonprofit organization that offers groups and programs for children who have a parent diagnosed with cancer. They provide answers to questions about cancer, support for children with a parent affected by cancer, an information packet with books and information specific to the needs of each child, referrals to local groups with monthly meetings, a quarterly newsletter for children, summer camps, socials, and grief workshops. They also have a program called, "Teddy Bear Outreach," which is designed to help young children after a parent has been diagnosed.

Hospice Net
401 Bowling Avenue, Suite 51
Nashville, TN 37205-5124
Web site: *http://www.hospicenet.org*

Description: Hospice Net is an independent nonprofit organization that works exclusively through the Internet. It contains more than one hundred articles regarding end-of-life issues. Hospice nurses, social workers, bereavement counselors, and chaplains are available to answer questions via email. The web site includes information for patients and caregivers about hospice care, information about grief and loss, and a hospice locator service.

I Can Cope
American Cancer Society
1599 Clifton Road, NE
Atlanta, GA 30329-4251
Toll-free: 800-ACS-2345
Web site: *http://www2.cancer.org/bcn/cope.html*

Description: This program addresses the educational and psychological needs of people with cancer and their families. A series of eight classes discusses the disease, coping with daily health problems, controlling cancer-related pain, nutrition for the person with cancer, expressing feelings, living with limitations, and local resources. Through lectures, group discussions, and study assignments, the course helps people with cancer regain a sense of control over their lives.

Leukemia & Lymphoma Society (LLS)

600 Third Avenue
New York, NY 10011
Toll-free: 800-955-4572
Fax: 212-573-8925
Web site: *http://www.leukemia.org*

Description: Patient service programs and resources available through local chapters of the LLS include financial assistance, support groups, one-to-one volunteer visitors (in some chapters), patient education and information, and referral to local resources in the community.

Look Good...Feel Better (LGFB)

American Cancer Society (ACS)
Cosmetic, Toiletry and Fragrance
  Association Foundation (CTFA)
National Cosmetology Association (NCA)
Toll-free: 800-395-LOOK
Web site: *http://www.lookgoodfeelbetter.org*
Web site: *http://www.lookgoodfeelbetter
  .org/index_7.00.html* (Spanish version)

Description: In partnership with the CTFA, the NCA, and the ACS, this free public service program is designed to teach women with cancer beauty techniques to help restore their appearance and self-image during chemotherapy and radiation treatment. *Information is also available in Spanish.*

Make Today Count

Mid-American Cancer Center
1235 East Cherokee
Springfield, MO 65804-2263
Toll-free: 800-432-2273
Phone: 417-885-2273
Fax: 417-888-8761

Description: Support organization for people affected by cancer or other life-threatening illness.

Man to Man

American Cancer Society
1599 Clifton Road, NE
Atlanta, GA 30329-4251
Toll-free: 800-ACS-2345
Web site: *http://www.cancer.org*

Description: Man to Man is a prostate cancer education and support program that offers community based group education, discussion and support to men with prostate cancer.

National Coalition for Cancer Survivorship (NCCS)

1010 Wayne Avenue
Silver Spring, MD 20910
Toll-free: 888-937-6227
Phone: 301-650-8868 or
  301-565-8195 (for publications)
Fax: 301-565-9670
Web site: *http://www.cansearch.org*
Web site: *http://www.cansearch.org/
  spanish/index.html* (Spanish version)

Description: The NCCS is a network of independent organizations working in the area of cancer survivorship and support. The web site offers links to on-line cancer resources, support groups, survivorship programs, the Cancer Survival Toolbox™, and newsletter.

National Family Caregivers Association (NFCA)

10605 Concord Street, Suite 501
Kensington, MD 20895-2504
Toll-free: 800-896-3650
Fax: 301-942-2302
Web site: *http://www.nfcacares.org*
Publication: *The Resourceful Caregiver from the National Family Caregivers Association.*

Description: NFCA is a national organization that focuses on family caregivers. It offers information and education, support, public awareness, and advocacy.

National Hospice Organization (NHO)

1901 N. Moore Street, Suite 901
Arlington, VA 22209
Hospice Helpline: 800-658-8898
Phone: 703-243-5900
Fax: 703-525-5762
Web site: *http://www.nho.org*

Description: NHO provides information about hospice programs in local areas and other publications. They also offer a discussion forum on their web site and other related links.

Reach to Recovery

American Cancer Society
1599 Clifton Road, NE
Atlanta, GA 30329-4251
Toll-free: 800-ACS-2345
Web site: *http://www.cancer.org*

Description: This program is designed to help patients with breast cancer cope with their diagnosis, treatment, and recovery. The volunteers from this program are women who have had breast cancer and are specially trained to share their knowledge and experiences in a supportive and nonintrusive manner. Ongoing support groups are available to help deal with the challenges of breast cancer. Reach to Recovery also provides early support to women who may have breast cancer or have just been diagnosed with cancer.

Well Spouse Foundation

30 East 40th Street
New York, NY 10018
Toll-free: 800-838-0879
Phone: 212-685-8815
Fax: 212-685-8676
Web site: *http://www.wellspouse.org*

Description: The Well Spouse Foundation is a national organization that provides support to partners of the chronically ill and/or disabled. They offer letter writing support groups, a bi-monthly newsletter, annual conferences, and weekend meetings. They also make referrals to local support groups throughout the country. The organization is involved with other groups in educating health care professionals, politi-

cians, and the public about the needs of "well spouses," and the importance of long-term care.

Wellness Community

35 East Seventh Street, Suite 412
Cincinnati, OH 45202-2420
Toll-free: 888-793-9355
Phone: 513-421-7111
Fax: 513-421-7119
Web site: *http://www.wellness-community.org*

Description: The Wellness Community is a nonprofit organization whose mission is to help people with cancer and their families enhance their health and well being by providing a professional program of emotional support, education, and hope. Support groups are facilitated by licensed counselors. Bereavement support groups are also available. Referrals are provided to their 25 facilities across the nation. The web site has information about relaxation, talking with children when a parent has cancer, and a study sponsored by the Wellness Community investigating the benefits of a professionally facilitated, online support group for women with breast cancer.

Y-Me National Breast Cancer Organization

212 West Van Buren
Chicago, IL 60607
Toll-free hotline: 800-221-2141
Toll-free hotline (Spanish): 800-986-9505
Phone: 312-986-8338
Fax: 312-294-8598
Web site: *http://www.y-me.org*
Web site: *http://www.y-me.org/spanish.htm* (*Spanish version*)

Description: This organization focuses on providing information and support to people with breast cancer and their families. Y-Me provides a national hotline, public meetings and seminars, workshops for professionals, referral services, support groups, a newsletter, a resource library, a teen program, and advocacy information.

Professional
Mental Health Organizations

American Association for Marriage and Family Therapy (AAMFT)

1133 15th Street, NW, Suite 300
Washington, DC 20005-2710
Phone: 202-452-0109
Fax: 202-223-2329
Web site: *http://www.aamft.org*

Description: This organization provides referrals to local marriage and family therapists. They also provide educational materials on helping couples live with illness and other issues related to families and health.

American Association of Pastoral Counselors

9504-A Lee Highway
Fairfax, VA 22031-2303
Toll-free: 800-225-5603
Phone: 703-385-6967
Web site: *http://www.aapc.org*

Description: This organization provides an online directory of Certified Pastoral Counselors across the country.

American Counseling Association (ACA)

5999 Stevenson Avenue
Alexandria, VA 22304-3300
Toll-free: 800-347-6647
Phone: 703-823-9800
Fax: 703-823-0252
Web site: *http://www.counseling.org/ consumers_media*

Description: The ACA provides information in the field of counseling and public fact sheets on coping with crisis. They also provide information about how to locate a professional counselor through the National Board of Certified Counselors (http://www. nbcc.org/consumer.htm) and other sources.

American Psychiatric Association

1400 K Street, NW
Washington, DC 20005
Toll-free: 888-357-7924
Fax: 202-682-6850

Web site: *http://www.psych.org*
Description: This organization provides information on mental health and referrals.

American Psychological Association (APA)

750 First Street, NE
Washington, DC 20002-4242
Toll-free: 800-964-2000
 (public education information line)
Toll-free: 800-374-2721
 (general information)
Phone: 202-336-5500
Web site: *http://www.apa.org*

Description: The APA offers referrals to psychologists in local areas. They also provide information on family issues, parenting, and health. The APA has links to state psychological associations that may also provide local referrals.

International Society of Psychiatric-Mental Health Nurses (ISPN)

1211 Locust Street
Philadelphia, PA 19107
Toll-free: 800-826-2950
Fax: 215-545-8107
Web site: *http://www.ispn-psych.org*

Description: The ISPN consists of specialty psychiatric-mental health nurses who treat patients with medical and mental health issues through counseling and education.

National Association of Social Workers (NASW)

750 First Street, NE, Suite 700
Washington, DC 20002-4241
Toll-free: 800-638-8799
Phone: 202-408-8600
Web site: *http://www.naswdc.org*

Description: This organization is concerned with advocacy, work practice standards and ethics, and professional standards for agencies employing social workers. The web site provides a national register of clinical social workers for local referrals.

Cancer Information

American Cancer Society (ACS)
1599 Clifton Road, NE
Atlanta, GA 30329-4251
Toll-free: 800-ACS-2345
Web site: *http://www.cancer.org*

Description: The ACS is the nationwide, community-based, voluntary health organization dedicated to eliminating cancer as a major health problem by preventing cancer, saving lives, and diminishing suffering from cancer through research, education, advocacy, and service. The ACS provides educational material and information on cancer, maintains several patient programs, directs people to services in their community including workshops and support groups, and provides funding for research.

American Medical Association (AMA)
515 North State Street
Chicago, IL 60610
Toll-free: 800-262-3211
Phone: 312-464-5000
Web site: *http://www.ama-assn.org*

Description: The AMA develops and promotes standards in medical practice, research, and education. Under the consumer health information section, the web site contains databases on physicians and hospitals, which can be searched by medical specialty. A pull-down menu of specific conditions is also provided.

American Society for Therapeutic Radiology and Oncology (ASTRO)
12500 Fair Lakes Circle, Suite 375
Fairfax, VA 22033-3882
Toll-free: 800-962-7876
Phone: 703-502-1550
Fax: 703-502-7852
Web site: *http://www.astro.org*

Description: Focusing on the use of radiation therapy for the treatment of cancer, this society's web site includes an overview of radiation therapy and a list of frequently asked questions.

American Society of Clinical Oncology (ASCO)
225 Reinekers Lane, Suite 650
Alexandria, VA 22314
Toll-free: 888-651-3038
Phone: 703-299-0150
Fax: 703-299-1044
Web site: *http://www.asco.org*

Description: The ASCO is an international medical society representing about 10,000 cancer specialists involved in clinical research and patient care. The ASCO web site is a resource for cancer patients, doctors, and researchers and includes patient guides, a glossary of cancer terms, an ASCO member oncologist locator, news and information about different cancers and drug treatments, information about cancer legislation, summaries of government reports, and links to related sites.

Association of Community Cancer Centers (ACCC)
11600 Nebel Street, Suite 201
Rockville, MD 20852-2557
Phone: 301-984-9496
Fax: 301-770-1949
Web site: *http://www.accc-cancer.org*

Description: This national organization includes over 600 medical centers, hospitals, and cancer programs. This web site contains a searchable database of cancer centers listed by state as well as information about oncology drugs (registration is required), and specific cancers.

Cancer Research Institute (CRI)
681 Fifth Avenue
New York, NY 10022
Toll-free: 800-992-2623
Phone: 212-688-7515
Fax: 212-832-9376
Web site: *http://www.cancerresearch.org*

Description: An institute funding cancer research and providing public information on cancer immunology and cancer treatment, the CRI helps locate immunotherapy clinical trials, and offers a cancer reference guide and other informational booklets.

CANCERLIT (Bibliographic Database)
Web site: *http://cnetdb.nci.nih.gov/cancerlit.html*

Description: This searchable site is maintained by the NCI and contains cancer articles published in medical and scientific journals, books, government reports, and articles that were presented at national meetings. A link to the PDQ (CancerNet/NCI database) search engine is provided, which allows people to search for clinical trials by state, city, and type of cancer.

CancerTrials
Web site: *http://cancertrials.nci.nih.gov*

Description: Maintained by the NCI, this site offers information about on-going cancer clinical trials and explanations of what a trial is and what is involved. A link to the PDQ (CancerNet/NCI database) search engine is provided, which allows people to search for clinical trials by state, city, and type of cancer.

Centers for Disease Control and Prevention (CDC)
Toll-free: 888-842-6355
Web site: *http://www.cdc.gov/cancer/nbccedp*

Description: The toll-free number can be used to locate free or low-cost mammography and Pap test centers in local areas. The web site contains a searchable map of centers, information about breast cancer, downloadable publications, and links to related sources.

Mayo Clinic Online
Mayo Foundation for Medical Education and Research
Web site: *http://www.mayoclinic.com*

Description: This web site contains a database searchable by keyword and topic. It also offers questions and answers from Mayo Clinic specialists, as well as links to reference articles and cancer organizations.

Medscape
Web site: *http://www.medscape.com*

Description: Although registration is required to view some of the content, this web site offers a great deal of information on prescription drugs as well as medical articles. There are also links to several organizations, cancer centers, database and education web sites, journals, and government sites. The web site is also searchable by key word. Registration is free.

National Bone Marrow Transplant Link (NBMT Link)
20411 West 12 Mile Road, Suite 108
Southfield, MI 48076
Toll-free: 800-546-5268
Phone: 248-358-1886
Fax: 248-932-8483
Web site: *http://www.comnet.org/nbmtlink*

Description: Primarily serving as an information center for prospective bone marrow transplant patients, this site contains a BMT resource guide and a survivor's guide, both of which can be printed directly from a home computer. Resources for health care professionals are also available.

National Cancer Institute (NCI)
NCI Public Inquiries Office
Building 31, Room 10A03
31 Center Drive, MSC 2580
Bethesda, MD 20892-2580
Phone: 301-435-3848
Toll-free: 800-4-CANCER
Web site: *http://www.cancer.gov*

Description: This government agency provides cancer information through several services (see list below). NCI also offers information about FDA-certified mammography facilities in local areas through the toll-free number.

Cancer Information Service (CIS)
Web site: *http://cis.nci.nih.gov*

Description: The CIS provides information to consumers and health care professionals. The web site contains a wealth of information including pamphlets and brochures on cancer diagnosis, treatment, research, and prevention. The NCI also maintains a listing of current clinical trials and other resources that may be helpful. The NCI can also provide free pamphlets on various forms of cancer treatment, medication, clinical trials, and other cancer-related information. *Spanish speaking staff is available.*

CancerFax
Fax: 301-402-5874

Description: CancerFax includes information about cancer treatment, screening, prevention, and supportive care. To obtain a contents list, dial the fax number from a fax machine hand set and follow the recorded instructions.

CancerNet
Web site: *http://cancernet.nci.nih.gov*
Web site: *http://cancernet.nci.nih.gov/ sp_menu.htm* (*Spanish version*)
Web site (On-line ordering): *http://publications.nci.nih.gov*

Description: A comprehensive web site that contains information on diagnosis, treatment, support, resources, literature, clinical trials, prevention and risk factors, and testing. Up to 20 publications can be ordered on-line. The publications list is searchable. *Some publications are available in Spanish.*

National Center for Complementary and Alternative Medicine (NCCAM)
Web site: *http://altmed.od.nih.gov*

Description: This NIH web site provides information on some complementary and alternative methods being promoted to treat different diseases.

National Comprehensive Cancer Network (NCCN)
50 Huntingdon Pike, Suite 200
Rockledge, PA 19046
Toll-free: 800-909-NCCN
Phone: 215-728-4788
Fax: 215-728-3877
Web site: *http://www.nccn.org*

Description: The NCCN is a nonprofit organization that is an alliance of cancer centers. The American Cancer Society has partnered with NCCN to translate the NCCN Clinical Practice Guidelines into a patient-friendly resource. The guidelines offer easy to understand information for patients and family members about treatment options for each stage of cancer. The treatment guidelines for patients are available for breast, prostate, and colon and rectal cancer, as well as for nausea and vomiting, and cancer pain. More guidelines are currently being developed. Call ACS for the latest guidelines or view them online at either www.cancer.org or www.nccn.org.

National Library of Medicine (NLM) (includes MEDLINE)
Web site: *http://www.nlm.nih.gov*

Description: This NIH web site provides a search engine for health, medical, and scientific literature and research as well as links to other government resources.

NLM Gateway
Web site: *http://gateway.nlm.nih.gov/ gw/cmd*

Description: As part of the National Library of Medicine, this web site offers links to searchable databases and allows users to search simultaneously in multiple retrieval systems at the NLM.

PubMed
Web site: *http://www.ncbi.nlm.nih.gov/ PubMed*

Description: Also part of the National Library of Medicine, this site provides access to literature references in Medline and other databases, with links to on-line journals. The site is searchable by key word.

National Women's Health Information Center (NWHIC)
The Office on Women's Health
U.S. Department of Health and Human Services
8550 Arlington Boulevard, Suite 300

Fairfax, VA 22301
Toll-free: 800-994-9662
Fax: 703-560-6598
Web site: ***http://www.4woman.gov***
Web site: ***http://www.4woman.gov/
Spanish/index.htm*** (*Spanish version*)

Description: This web site has a searchable database of information on various women's health issues, including breast cancer. Documents accessible through this site include information from the NCI, the CDC, and several other government agencies. The site contains a section for special groups, which separates breast cancer and other health information by specific minority group. It also contains links to on-line medical dictionaries and journals.

***Self Help for Women with Breast or
Ovarian Cancer (SHARE)***
1501 Broadway, Suite 1720
New York, NY 10036
Phone (Hotline): 212-382-2111
Phone (Spanish Hotline): 212-719-4454
Fax: 212-869-3431
Web site: ***http://sharecancersupport.org***

Description: SHARE is a self-help organization that serves women who have been affected by breast cancer or ovarian cancer. Hotline volunteers are breast or ovarian cancer survivors. They provide information about breast cancer, emotional support, printed materials, and referrals to national organizations. Their web site includes information on the hotlines and support programs in New York City. *Spanish speaking staff available.*

Additional Reading
Pamphlets

After Diagnosis: A Guide for Patients and Families. Atlanta, Ga.: American Cancer Society, 800-ACS-2345 (www.cancer.org).

It Helps to Have Friends When Mom or Dad Has Cancer. Designed for the child whose mom or dad has cancer, this booklet addresses the importance of discussing thoughts and feelings with people the child knows and trusts. Atlanta, Ga.: American Cancer Society, 800-ACS-2345 (www.cancer.org).

Kids Worry Too. University of Nebraska Medical Center, Child Life Department, Room 4145, 600 South 42nd Street, Omaha, NE, 68198-2165; 402-559-6775.

What About Me? A booklet for teenage children of cancer patients, by Linda Leopold Strauss. 1986. Cancer Family Care, Inc., 7162 Reading Road, Suite 1050, Cincinnati, OH, 45237; 513-731-3346.

When Someone in Your Family Has Cancer. Bethesda Md.: National Cancer Institute, 800-4-CANCER (www.cancer.gov).

When Your Brother or Sister Has Cancer. Atlanta, Ga.: American Cancer Society, 800-ACS-2345 (www.cancer.org).

Books

FOR CHILDREN

Ackermann, A., and A. Ackermann. 2001. *Our Mom Has Cancer.* Atlanta, Ga.: American Cancer Society.

Boulden, J. 1995. *When Someone Is Very Sick.* Weaverville, Calif.: Boulden Publishing.

Carney, K. L. 1999. *What IS Cancer, Anyway? Explaining Cancer to Children of All Ages.* Wethersfield, Conn.: Dragonfly Publishing.

Fox Chase Cancer Center. 1998. *Kids' Night Out: A Journal for Families Dealing with Cancer.* Philadelphia: Fox Chase.

Ganz, P., and T. Scofield. 1996. *Life Isn't Always a Day At the Beach: A Book for All Children Whose Lives Are Affected By Cancer.* Lincoln, Nebr.: High Five Publishing.

Gelman, M., and T. Hartman. 1999. *Lost & Found: A Kid's Book for Living Through Loss.* New York: Morrow Junior Books.

Goodman, M. B. 1991. *Vanishing Cookies: Doing Okay When a Parent Has Cancer.* Ontario, Canada: The Benjamin Family Foundation, 416-663-9060.

Heiney, S., C. Howell, and E. Vinton. 1998. *Quest: A Journal for the Teenager Whose Parent Has Cancer.* Columbia, S.C.: South Carolina Cancer Center of the Palmetto Health Alliance.

Kohlenberg, S. 1993. *Sammy's Mom Has Cancer.* Washington, D.C.: Magination Press.

Mayer, M. 1992. *There's a Nightmare in My Closet.* New York: E. P. Dutton.

Navarra, T. 1989. *On My Own: Helping Kids Help Themselves.* New York: Barron's Educational Series, Inc.

Parkinson, C. S. 1991. *My Mommy Has Cancer.* New York: Park Press.

Steele, D. W., and H. E. King. 1995. *Kemo Shark.* Atlanta, Ga.: KidsCope, www.kidscope.org. A 16-page color "comic book" designed to help children with in a family where a parent has cancer and undergoes chemotherapy.

Vigna, J. 1993. *When Eric's Mom Fought Cancer.* Morton Grove, Ill.: Albert Whitman & Co.

Vogel, C. 1995. *Will I Get Breast Cancer? Questions and Answers for Teenage Girls.* Morristown, N.J.: Silver Burdett Press.

Winthrop, E., and B. Lewin. 2000. *Promises.* Boston, Mass.: Houghton Mifflin.

Yaffe, R. S., and T. Cramer. 1998. *Once Upon a Hopeful Night.* Pittsburgh, Pa.: Oncology Nursing Press.

FOR PARENTS

American Cancer Society. 2001. *A Breast Cancer Journey.* Atlanta, Ga.: American Cancer Society.

American Cancer Society. 2001. *American Cancer Society's Guide to Pain Control.* Atlanta, Ga.: American Cancer Society.

American Cancer Society. 2000. *American Cancer Society's Guide to Complementary and Alternative Cancer Methods.* Atlanta, Ga.: American Cancer Society.

Bostwick, D. G., G. T. MacLennan, and T. R. Larson. 1999. *Prostate Cancer: What Every Man—and His Family—Needs to Know.* Rev. ed. New York: Villard.

Davis, M., M. McKay, and E. R. Eshelman. 2000. *Relaxation and Stress Reduction Workbook.* Oakland, Ca.: New Harbinger Publications.

Eyre, H., D. Lange, and L. B. Morris. 2001. *Informed Decisions: The Complete Book of Cancer Diagnosis, Treatment, and Recovery, 2nd Ed.* Atlanta, Ga.: American Cancer Society.

Harpham, W. S. 1997. *When a Parent Has Cancer: A Guide to Caring for Your Children.* New York: Harper Collins. Includes *Becky and the Worry Cup*, an illustrated children's book that tells the story of a seven-year-old girl's experience with her mother's cancer. The child can read this book alone or together with a parent.

Hermann, J. F., S. L. Wojtkowiak, P. S. Houts, and S. B. Kahn. 1988. *Helping People Cope: A Guide for Families Facing Cancer.* Harrisburg, Pa.: Pennsylvania Department of Health, 800-722-2623 (www.oncolink.upenn.edu/psychosocial/books/cope).

Holland, J. C., and S. Lewis. 2000. *The Human Side of Cancer: Living with Hope, Coping with Uncertainty.* New York: HarperCollins.

Houts, P., and J. Bucher. 2000. *Caregiving: A Step-By-Step Resource for Caring for the Person with Cancer at Home.* Atlanta, Ga.: American Cancer Society.

Levin, B. 1999. *Colorectal Cancer: A Thorough and Compassionate Resource for Patients and Their Families.* New York: Villard.

McCue, K. 1994. *How to Help Children Through a Parent's Serious Illness.* New York: St. Martin's Press.

Runowicz, C. D., J. A. Petrek, and T. S. Gansler. 1999. *Women and Cancer: A Thorough and Compassionate Resource for Patients and Their Families.* New York: Villard.

Wilkes, G. M., T. B. Ades, and I. Krakoff. 2000. *Consumers Guide to Cancer Drugs.* Toronto: Jones & Bartlett.

Videotapes

Hear How I Feel. 1996. Young adults talk about their parents' cancer. 30 min. Northeastern Ontario Regional Cancer Centre, 705-5-CANCER (www.neorc.on.ca).

Kids Tell Kids What It Is Like When a Family Member Has Cancer. 1998. Interviews with children whose parents have cancer. 30 min. Cancervive, 310-203-9232 (www.cancervive.org).

My Mom Has Breast Cancer: A Guide for Families. 1996. Psychologist presents information and interviews with children. 33 min. KidsCope, (www.kidscope.org).

Talking About Your Cancer: A Parent's Guide to Helping Children Cope. 1996. Video for parents on talking to their children about their cancer. 18 min. Fox Chase Cancer Center, 215-728-2668 (www.fccc.edu).

When a Parent Has Cancer: Looney Professor Boonie Explains Cancer to Kids! Thunderbird Samaritan Medical Center, Oncology Social Work, 5555 West Thunderbird Road, Glendale, AZ, 85306; 602-588-5450 (www.bannerhealthaz.com/centers/thunderbird_sam.html).

INDEX

About the Authors

SUE P. HEINEY, PH.D., R.N., C.S., F.A.A.N., is the Manager of Psychosocial Oncology at South Carolina Cancer Center of Palmetto Health in Columbia, South Carolina. She has provided psychotherapy for patients and families since 1981. She is internationally recognized for her psychosocial expertise and has received the Lane W. Adams Award from the American Cancer Society, and the Excellence in Practice Award from Sigma Theta Tau International. In 1995, she presented the Mara Mogensen Flaherty Lectureship, the Healing Power of Story, for the Oncology Nursing Society. In 1998, she was inducted into the American Academy of Nursing.

JOAN F. HERMANN, M.S.W., L.S.W., is the Director of Social Work Services at Fox Chase Cancer Center in Philadelphia, Pennsylvania. Her background includes both pediatric and adult oncology. She was a founding member of the Association of Oncology Social Work and received its Leadership in Oncology Social Work Award in 1993. She also received the Distinguished Service Award from the American Cancer Society in 1994. She is a member of the editorial boards of the *Journal of Psychosocial Oncology, Cancer Practice,* and *Oncology Times.* She has authored numerous publications and has a special interest in the needs of children of adult cancer patients.

KATHERINE V. BRUSS, PSY.D., is the Managing Editor for book publishing at the American Cancer Society in Atlanta, Georgia. She is a licensed psychologist with 18 years of clinical experience. She has published over a dozen articles in academic journals and other university publications. She brings her psycho-oncology perspective to her current work, which she incorporates into materials for patients, families, caregivers, and professionals.

JOY L. FINCANNON, R.N., M.S., is an Associate Medical Editor at the American Cancer Society in Atlanta, Georgia. She is a psychiatric clinical nurse specialist with experience in working with cancer patients, their families, and cancer health professionals. Ms. Fincannon has published in nursing journals and medical textbooks, and has been a psychotherapist in private practice for many years.